Healthy Living with Diabetes

Margot Joan Fromer

New Harbinger Publications

Publisher's Note

This publication is designed to provide accurate and authoritative information in regard to the subject matter covered. It is sold with the understanding that the publisher is not engaged in rendering psychological, financial, legal, or other professional services. If expert assistance or counseling is needed, the services of a competent professional should be sought.

Distributed in the U.S.A. by Publishers Group West; in Canada by Raincoast Books; in Great Britain by Airlift Book Company, Ltd.; in South Africa by Real Books, Ltd.; in Australia by Boobook; and in New Zealand by Tandem Press.

New Harbinger Publications, Inc.
5674 Shattuck Avenue
Oakland, CA 94609

Cover design by Poulson/Gluck Design.
Edited by Angela Watrous.
Text design by Tracy Marie Powell.

Library of Congress Catalog Card Number: 97-95483.
ISBN 1-57224-112-8

Printed in the United States of America on recycled paper.

New Harbinger Publications' Web site address: www.newharbinger.com.

First printing

Contents

Introduction

On an early Friday evening in December, two days after a routine physical checkup and blood test, my doctor called. "Guess what," she said, cheerfully and with no preamble. "You have diabetes. Your blood sugar is over three hundred."

Just like that. Wham, out of the blue.

I was instructed to make an appointment with a diabetes educator in her office who would teach me how to take care of myself and how to go on a diabetic diet. That was it. The conversation lasted no more than two minutes. There were no expressions of sympathy for a patient who had suddenly come down with a serious illness, no apology for imparting such shocking and unexpected news in such an abrupt manner, no comfort that things would not be nearly as bad as they now seemed, no assurance that if I did indeed take care of myself, I would probably live to a ripe old age.

I hung up the phone and sat, stunned, at the dining room table where I had been about to eat dinner. For once, my appetite completely disappeared, and as I shoved the plate away, my mind was filled with images of all the disastrous things that could happen as a result of diabetes.

Because I am both a nurse and a medical writer, the images were plentiful and graphic. I have a good imagination and was scared out of my wits, so those fantasies were dripping with disaster and tragedy. I saw myself going blind and having a bad heart and no legs—that is, if I lived long enough to sink into the worst complications diabetes has to offer. I put my head down on the table and sobbed—and resolved to kill myself if I lost my sight or my feet, or if I had a heart attack.

When the tears subsided, I reached for the phone to call a few friends to tell them what had happened to me—and to get some sympathy. But I pulled my hand back. I didn't want to tell anyone that I had diabetes. When I realized why I was reluctant to make those calls, I broke into a fresh onslaught of tears. I was ashamed.

I felt as though I had brought it on myself: by letting my sweet tooth get the best of me on more occasions than I was willing to admit even to myself, by being a "lazy slob" and refusing to exercise, by refusing to switch to low-fat foods and not eating enough fruits and vegetables, by being what I considered a thoroughly bad person—at least in terms of what I put in my mouth. The fact that I don't smoke, that I drink a negligible amount of alcohol, and that my genetic endowment probably played a key role in my having diabetes was not a comfort. Not when I was so intent on being as miserable as possible.

A year and a half later, as I sit at my computer writing these words, I am healthier than I have been in a decade. I feel fine. My blood sugar is a little high, but it is well within normal limits for a diabetic. I've lost more than fifty pounds, and I'm actually looking forward to my daily exercise, a three-mile walk, this afternoon.

How did I progress from frantic fear and despair to feeling great and being glad to be alive? The same way you are going to do it: by learning about diabetes, by acknowledging all the really scary feelings that it engenders, and by slowly but surely teaching yourself how to live with the disease and incorporate it into your (much healthier) lifestyle so that you are not engulfed by constant feelings of deprivation and depression.

You are not alone, not by a long shot. Between fourteen and sixteen million Americans are living with the disease, 90 percent of whom have Type II diabetes. A half million more are diagnosed each year.

You will always have diabetes. It is an incurable disease. But it is highly controllable, and you will learn to control it. If you are one of the vast majority of diabetics who have Type II diabetes (non-insulin-dependent diabetic), and if you have contracted it as an adult (the most common time of onset), it is highly unlikely that you will have to take medication.

Diabetes is a serious illness—the seventh-leading cause of death in the United States and the single leading cause of kidney disease. More than 250,000 Americans die each year from complications of diabetes. The disease is also the leading cause of blindness and, aside from traumatic injury, the chief cause of amputations in the United States.

Therefore, you must take it seriously. But it need not rule your life. You do not have to think about every morsel of food that passes your lips, and if you choose not to, there is no reason why you have to tell people you are a diabetic.

You can eat in restaurants (even an occasional fast-food joint), you can share meals with friends in their homes, you can go on business trips, and no one but you need know that you are on a "special" diet. Because a diabetic diet is really no more special than the ordinary diet of someone who is trying to eat sensibly and adhere to the guidelines of good nutrition.

Your exercise regimen won't be special either—at least no more so than anyone who is trying to shed a few pounds and tone up their muscles, and that's practically everyone these days. You don't have to go to the gym to pump iron, and you need not turn into a sweat-drenched jock. But you might buy yourself a bicycle or learn the hiking trails near your home, or you might sign up for an aerobics class or join the local swim club, and you'll be doing exactly what your friends and co-workers do—having fun while getting in shape.

And there is more good news: Many of the complications of diabetes, as well as the defects underlying the illness, can be controlled and treated—particularly in the type of diabetes that develops in adults.

As you read *Healthy Living with Diabetes*, you will notice a major recurring theme: control. That is the key to living a long, healthy, and happy life as a diabetic. You will learn to:

- Control the disease so it doesn't control you
- Understand and cope with your feelings about diabetes
- Change your lifestyle in ways that will benefit your general health as well as help keep your diabetes under control
- Learn easy and practical tips for exercising gently but effectively
- Test your own blood glucose level and learn the factors that affect it

- Follow guidelines for the way diabetics (and everyone, for that matter) ought to eat
- Correctly take whatever medication you might need, either permanently or temporarily
- Prevent health problems that can accompany diabetes

1

Diabetes: An Overview

Diabetes mellitus is the full and correct name for the disease, but most people, doctors included, call it diabetes. Descriptions of the disease have been found in the annals of ancient Egyptian, Indian, Arabic, and Chinese medicine. The word "diabetes" comes from the Greek, meaning "to flow through," and mellitus comes from the Latin and means "honeyed." Therefore, diabetes mellitus describes a condition in which sugar (which we now call glucose) appears in the urine.

Over the centuries, diabetes was treated with a variety of methods to lower the sugar content of the urine (which was determined by smelling it), almost all of which involved what the patient ate or didn't eat. Some patients were told to feast and fast on alternate weeks, others were given rancid meat to eat. Vegetables cooked three times in their own water was popular for a while, as was a diet consisting only of grains and eggs. Despite various treatments, the association of food with diabetes has been there since the beginning.

A diagnosis of diabetes was almost always a death sentence, usually within a year or two after onset. Even now, if the disease is left unchecked and uncontrolled, it is fatal. But now there is a way to control it. In 1860, the German physician Paul Langerhans discovered that groups of cells in the pancreas (a gland near the stomach) produce insulin, a hormone that metabolizes glucose. This discovery paved the way for two Canadian researchers, Frederick Banting and Charles Best, to experiment with injecting insulin into dogs with diabetes. Their efforts were so successful that they felt emboldened to give insulin to human beings. The treatment greatly improved the lives, as well as the life expectancy, of diabetics.

Oral hypoglycemic agents (drugs that lower blood glucose) were introduced in the early 1960s. The first convenient-to-use urine test was developed at the end of World War II, and in 1980, people were able to monitor their own blood glucose levels at home. In 1994, a ten-year nationwide study called the Diabetes Control and Complications Trial (NIDDK), which involved thousands of people, proved that keeping tight control over blood glucose levels prevents, delays, or lessens the severity of the major complications of diabetes.

Not all diabetes is caused by the inability of the islets of Langerhans (named after the physician who discovered the cells) in the pancreas to produce sufficient amounts of the hormone known as insulin. Some people with diabetes have normal insulin levels, but the insulin does not efficiently metabolize glucose. This is known as Type II diabetes; the former is called Type I.

Although there are exceptions, people with Type I diabetes need to take insulin, and those with Type II do not. For this reason, Type I is called insulin-dependent diabetes, and Type II is called non-insulin-dependent diabetes. However, most diabetics and their physicians call it Type I and Type II and that is what I do in this book.

Causes and Mechanisms of Diabetes

Almost all the food people eat is digested and converted into a substance called glucose, one of the many chemical formulations of sugar (among the others are fructose, lactose, and sucrose). Glucose provides the energy needed by the body to maintain all its functions: from jumping high hurdles to sitting quietly and thinking. Glucose is absolutely essential for cell function. Without it, the cell dies. When too many essential cells die, the entire body dies.

Food is digested and acted upon by insulin and converted into glucose, which enters the bloodstream from the digestive tract and is taken up by every single cell in the body. On the wall of each cell is a structure called an insulin receptor, which indicates when and how much glucose the cell needs. The cell then absorbs glucose from the bloodstream and either uses it immediately to provide energy or stores it for later use. The amount of glucose in the bloodstream is controlled by the action of insulin (which in turn is regulated by the cells' insulin receptors), and when the two substances work in harmony, all is well: the pancreas responds to the food you eat and releases the precise amount of insulin needed to correctly use the glucose from the food.

Blood glucose levels fluctuate, in part, according to what and when you have eaten. For instance, if you eat a lot of simple carbohydrates (sweet desserts, doughnuts, pastry, lots of sugar in your coffee or tea), your blood glucose level will soar very quickly and will return to normal soon. If you eat excessively over long periods of time, no matter what the food, your blood glucose level will stay high. If you eat less, your levels will decrease.

By the same token, the more physically active you are, the more glucose leaves the bloodstream and enters the cells to provide energy; therefore, your blood glucose level will be lower. If you exercise strenuously over a short period of time, causing your cells to require large amounts of glucose for energy, they will soon use up what is currently in your bloodstream and you will have insufficient blood glucose (hypoglycemia). If you exercise less rigorously over a longer period of time, your body will obtain glucose from where it is stored in fat cells and use it for fuel, and you will eventually lose weight.

Under these normal conditions, the islets of Langerhans produce sufficient insulin. However, in diabetes, too much glucose remains in the bloodstream and spills over into the urine. This can happen for three different reasons: the islets of Langerhans produce too little insulin, there are too few insulin receptor sites in the cells, or once the insulin attaches to a receptor site, its signal does not get through to the cell (a condition called insulin resistance).

No one knows the precise cause of diabetes, although the *tendency* toward the disease is inherited. In this case, lack of exercise, high levels of stress, and being overweight might cause someone to develop Type II disease (Type I has little to do with these factors).

Another possible causative factor is exposure to certain chemicals: Vacor (a rat poison), Pentamidine chemotherapy (used to treat pneumonia), and L-asparaginase (used in cancer chemotherapy). These agents, combined with a genetic predisposition to diabetes, could increase risk—or even cause the disease (Atkinson and Maclaren 1994).

Whatever the cause, diabetics have too much glucose in their bloodstream and too little in their cells. This results in a lack of energy, which is why you probably feel tired and washed out when your glucose level is too high. And if you feel pooped, imagine the effect on your highly glucose-sensitive organs such as your heart, blood vessels, nerves, eyes, kidneys, and brain.

Diabetes is a progressive disease, which means that if it is not controlled, it will do more and more damage to your body over time. Eventually, if you do nothing, it will kill you But at the same time, it is highly controllable, and if you take the appropriate steps to keep your blood glucose levels within normal limits, you will be able to avoid most or all of the negative health consequences of the disease.

Types of Diabetes

Type I Diabetes

In Type I (insulin-dependent) diabetes, the pancreas stops making insulin because the insulin-producing cells have been destroyed, probably by one's own immune system. This is what is known as an autoimmune disease. Type I diabetes used to be called juvenile diabetes because its age of onset is earlier than Type II: usually before age thirty. However, anyone of any age can develop Type I diabetes.

Current medical thinking says that the malfunction in the immune system may originate with a genetic defect and be triggered into action by a viral infection. In the process of fighting the virus, the immune system somehow goes into "overdrive" and is unable to shut itself off when all the viruses have been killed. It goes on to attack healthy cells, including insulin-producing ones in the pancreas. Eventually, all these cells are destroyed and the pancreas can no longer produce insulin. In general, at the time of diagnosis, people with Type I are often very thin and have high levels of ketones in their urine.

Type II Diabetes

Type II (non-insulin-dependent) diabetes occurs most commonly in people over age forty who are overweight and may have high blood pressure (hypertension) and high blood cholesterol. Type II diabetics have few or no ketones in their urine at diagnosis. With Type II, the pancreas produces insulin, but the insulin does not work efficiently. The cells send a signal back to the pancreas, which in turn senses a too-high blood glucose level. The pancreas then manufactures more and more insulin in an effort to move the glucose from the bloodstream into the cells. Over the years, the pancreas may exhaust itself and stop producing insulin, in which case you would have to take insulin injections. But this last-ditch effort by the pancreas is rare in Type II diabetes.

Some people believe that Type II diabetes is not as serious as Type I because Type II may not require taking insulin. For this reason, they may treat it lightly, ignore dietary suggestions, and believe that their illness is "nothing." This isn't true, and it's dangerous to treat diabetes lightly.

Gestational Diabetes

Gestational diabetes occurs only during pregnancy when a woman's body cannot manufacture sufficient insulin to accommodate natural hormonal changes. Pregnant women may need two to three times the amount of insulin that nonpregnant women require. All women should be tested for gestational diabetes between the twenty-fourth and twenty-sixth weeks of pregnancy.

Gestational diabetes may be caused by one or more of the following factors: various hormones produced by the placenta that block the action of insulin; a genetic predisposition similar to Type II diabetes; and obesity in the prepregnant state.

Gestational diabetes disappears after birth, but the woman will always have a higher-than-average risk of developing Type II diabetes in later life. If the gestational diabetes is actually Type II diabetes that simply was not diagnosed until pregnancy, it will not disappear after birth. If a woman has had gestational diabetes, she should have her blood glucose checked by a physician at least once a year for the rest of her life. Gestational diabetes is treated in the same way as Type II, although if it is severe, insulin injections might be required.

Diabetes Risk Factors

Because the symptoms of diabetes are varied and can be elusive, it is important to identify people at highest risk for the disease. They should have regular medical checkups to catch the disease early before major damage occurs.

Obese people carry an unusually high risk of Type II diabetes. In fact, 60 to 90 percent of people with this form of the disease are overweight. Studies sponsored by the U.S. Public Health Service show that among the Pima Indians of the southwestern United States, the ethnic group with the highest known incidence of Type II diabetes in the world, obesity is a major health problem. Moreover, the Public Health Service estimates that one in three Americans is obese, which will increase the incidence of the disease as these people age.

With few exceptions, Americans eat too much and have generally poor diets that are too high in fat and simple sugars. As the percentage of Americans with these risk factors increases, the percentage of Americans with diabetes also will increase, creating the distinct possibility that diabetes will become the most common serious chronic disease in the United States.

The risk for Type II diabetes for both sexes increases with age. As the body ages, its ability to efficiently use insulin begins to deteriorate. Older people who are overweight and who live a sedentary lifestyle are especially prone to diabetes, and they are more likely than younger Type II diabetics to require medication. An estimated 23 percent of all people age sixty-five to seventy have impaired glucose tolerance. This tends to worsen over time, so the incidence of overt (but perhaps not diagnosed) diabetes in people age eighty and older may be as high as 40 percent.

Heredity is another risk factor. In Type I, generally you need to inherit genetic susceptibility from both parents, but because most people who are at risk do not get diabetes, there must be other factors at work. Researchers are looking at a number of environmental influences: long-term exposure to cold weather; viruses; and diet in early life, especially the role of breast feeding.

Type II diabetes has an even stronger genetic basis, but risk also is influenced by environmental factors. A family history of diabetes seems to play the strongest role among Americans and Europeans living a Western lifestyle: too much dietary fat and too little carbohydrates and fiber, as well as too little exercise.

Here are the statistics for the risk of the child of a diabetic getting diabetes—but remember statistics are only estimates of probability, not a statement of whether or not a child will inherit diabetes. In Type I, the odds of the child of a man with the disease getting it are one in seventeen. In a woman who delivered before age twenty-five, the risk of passing on the disease is one in twenty-five; if she delivered after age twenty-five, the risk is one in one hundred. If a woman developed diabetes before age eleven, the risk of her child having it is doubled. If both parents have Type I diabetes, the risk of a child also having it is between one in ten and one in four (Culverwell 1995).

If you have Type II, the risk of your child getting diabetes is one in seven if you were diagnosed before age fifty and one in thirteen if you were diagnosed after age fifty. Some scientists think that the risk is greater when the parent with diabetes is the mother. If both parents have Type II diabetes, the risk of a child inheriting it is about one in two (Culverwell 1995).

Symptoms and Diagnosis

Some diabetics have no symptoms at all, and the disease is discovered as a result of a routine blood test. In other cases, the symptoms are glaringly obvious: unexplained weight loss and increased thirst, hunger, and frequency of urination.

Most times, however, the "fuzzier" symptoms of diabetes (fatigue, lack of energy, irritability, blurred vision, frequent infections, numbness or tingling in the feet and, in women, unexplained vaginal yeast infections) are slow to develop, insidious, and may also be the symptoms of other illnesses.

Unfortunately, about 20 percent of diabetics already have signs of complications, especially eye and kidney problems, when they are diagnosed. In fact, it is these problems that may have prompted testing glucose level in the first place. Contrary to popular belief, there is no such thing as "just a slight touch" of diabetes or "borderline" diabetes. It's like pregnancy: you either have it or you don't.

Diabetes is diagnosed by measuring blood glucose. This is done in one of two ways. The first is by a test called *random* (or *casual*) blood glucose, in which the blood is drawn and tested at any time of day. If the result is 200 milligrams per deciliter (mg/dl) or higher, you have diabetes. A fasting blood glucose is drawn first thing in the morning, when you have not eaten anything for ten to twelve hours. Diabetes is diagnosed if the result is 140 mg/dl or higher on at least two separate occasions. A task force of the American Diabetes Association recently recommended dropping the level to 126 mg/dl.

The sooner diabetes is diagnosed the better, because early treatment and tight control results in fewer complications down the road. Because so many people don't know they have diabetes, the ADA task force also recommends annual diabetes screening for all adults over age forty-five.

Treatment

All diabetes treatment is aimed at one thing: controlling the level of glucose in the bloodstream. There are a variety of ways to do this, all of which depend on a number of factors: type of diabetes, age at onset, severity of symptoms and glucose level, presence of complicating factors, general health and current lifestyle, and the changes the diabetic is willing to make.

The three major categories of treatment are diet, exercise, and medication. In Type II diabetes, diet and exercise alone are often all that is necessary to bring blood glucose down to manageable levels. Sometimes oral medication is necessary. Type I diabetes is treated with insulin in addition to diet and exercise.

Oral hypoglycemic agents help the body metabolize the glucose obtained from food. These drugs are not insulin, but they do stimulate insulin-producing cells to secrete more insulin, and they help overcome insulin resistance.

Insulin injections, which you learn to give to yourself with a variety of implements, may be combined with an oral hypoglycemic agent, but usually a diabetic who needs insulin takes only insulin. This hormone used to be manufactured from pork and beef, but now most of it is genetically engineered and synthesized, which makes it identical to naturally occurring human insulin, thus more effective in treating human diabetes. See chapter 5 for a thorough discussion of medications to treat diabetes.

Controlling blood cholesterol and blood pressure also are important components of treatment. See chapter 3 for ways you can accomplish this with your diet.

Myths and Misconceptions

Of all the major chronic diseases that affect Americans, diabetes, which many people erroneously call "sugar diabetes," seems to be the one most surrounded by myth and misinformation. Following are some of the mistakes that people make about it, followed by the actual facts about the disease.

- *Diabetes is contagious.* No, it isn't. You probably inherited a genetic tendency to become diabetic, and may pass it on to your children, but you didn't "catch" it, nor can you "give" it to others.
- *You get diabetes from eating too much sugar.* No, you don't. Sugar itself does not cause the disease, although it certainly has an effect on blood glucose levels.
- *The medications your doctor gives you will cure the diabetes.* No, they won't. Research scientists are hard at work on a cure, but one has not yet been found. Blood glucose levels can be controlled and brought to near-normal levels with diet, exercise, and medications, but the disease itself is not cured.
- *The disease will go away by itself eventually.* No, it won't. Even if you have no symptoms (and with Type II diabetes, you may not have had any even when you were diagnosed), you still have diabetes, and you still need to work at controlling it. And even when your symptoms disappear because your diabetes is well-controlled, you still have the disease.
- *Type I diabetes is worse than Type II, and Type II can turn into Type I if you don't take care of yourself.* Neither is true. Although they have some things in common, Type I and Type II diabetes are two separate conditions.
- *I have just a "slight touch" of diabetes. I won't worry about it.* Wrong. You either have diabetes or you don't. If you do, you are a full-fledged diabetic and you need to treat it.
- *Diabetics are sickly people and you can't expect them to do a lot of physical things.* No, they're not. In fact, diabetics who have their disease in good control are usually more physically fit than the average person.
- *Diabetics can never touch alcohol.* Yes, they can, in moderation.
- *A diabetic woman who gets pregnant is asking for trouble; she could die.* Pregnant diabetics have the same chance of getting through the pregnancy in good shape and delivering a healthy baby as nondiabetics.

2

Immediate Physical and Emotional Needs

Once you find out that you are diabetic, there are some things you must attend to almost immediately. (By the way, while some people do not like the word "diabetic" and prefer to think of themselves as a "person with diabetes," I use "diabetic" in this book because one word is far smoother than three.)

Monitoring Blood Glucose

The first thing you have to do is start lowering your blood glucose levels. The most important aspect of diabetes care is keeping your blood glucose levels within a normal range for diabetics: 80–140 mg/dl fasting or 100–180 mg/dl one or two hours after meals. For nondiabetics, the numbers should be slightly lower: 75–115 mg/dl fasting and below 140 mg/dl after meals.

Everyone's blood glucose (diabetics and nondiabetics alike) fluctuates a good deal during the day, depending on how long it's been since you've eaten, what you ate for your last meal or snack, what medications you are taking, how much stress you're experiencing, how physically active you are during the day, and whether you have an illness such as a cold or the flu. The best way to keep your blood glucose on an even keel and within normal limits is to keep all these factors in balance. This book will teach you how to do that. There are three general steps in the process: testing your blood glucose, adjusting what you eat and drink and how much exercise you get, and retesting your blood to see how you are doing.

Testing Your Blood

No, you don't have to become a laboratory technician, and you don't have to wrap a tourniquet around your arm and stick a needle into your vein. Testing your own blood couldn't be any easier, and it's all practically automatic. Although a needle (often called a lancet) does prick your finger, you don't have to do the jabbing; all you do is press a button and the needle shoots out of the spring-loaded stylus automatically, and it's all over before you have a chance to get anxious. In fact, in a very short time, you will become so used to testing your own blood that you probably won't think of it as being pricked by a needle.

Your doctor or other health care provider (a diabetes educator or nurse practitioner) will have you buy a self blood glucose monitor (SBGM), which you can find in large drugstores and some supermarkets and discount stores. They come with a supply of test strips and needles, which you will have to replenish from time to time. There are a number of brands on the market. Although the design of the case varies from brand to brand, most function in about the same way and their inner workings and costs are similar. Many have rebate offers, so make sure you look at all the brands before you buy. Mine ended up costing only fifteen dollars after the rebate.

Just as you can spend more for a car if you want lots of options, you can spend more for a monitor that has a variety of bells and whistles. You can buy expensive laser technology or a more costly monitor with a reusable instead of disposable tests strips. Some work by electrical signal instead of a chemically treated test strip, and others even have a voice that tells you what your blood glucose level is. All monitors have a memory that tells you what your last test was, but more expensive models have long-term memory and written printouts. Others have the finger-piercing device built into the machine, rather than having to use a separate instrument. One costly system, called the DIVA, has a memory that stores up to three thousand events, including blood glucose, insulin dose, food intake, and exercise. The choice is up to you. You have to test your blood glucose, and you need a good, serviceable monitor to do it. Your monitor (at least a basic one) and all blood glucose testing supplies are tax deductible, so keep your receipts.

Your doctor will tell you how often to test your blood, but in the beginning, it will be several times a day at about the same hours. Yes, it's a bit of a nuisance at first, but again, you will quickly become used to the routine and will find that you have incorporated it into your life in much the same way as you brush your teeth or wash your face in the morning. You do it without thinking much about it.

Each time you test your blood glucose, write down the result, along with how long it has been since you ate and any other little notes you think are pertinent, such as the fact that you just finished exercising or that you had a fight with someone that morning. Your monitor will come with a booklet for this purpose, so keep the booklet with the machine and you won't feel as though you have added another paperwork chore to your life. The record gives you an opportunity to keep track of how you are doing with diabetes control, and it helps you correlate your diet and physical activity with your blood glucose level. You should bring the booklet with you each time you visit your physician so it can be checked.

It is extremely important to read the directions carefully before you begin using your SBGM. Read every word and keep the instruction booklet with the monitor. In general, however, this is the procedure:

1. Wash your hands thoroughly with soap and water. Warm water will increase the blood flow to your finger. Don't swab your skin with alcohol because it can interfere with the accuracy of the test. If your hands are cold, rub them together briskly to warm them.

2. Turn on the monitor and do what it tells you. First it will give you the reading from your last test, then it will tell you to insert the test strip in the appropriate slot and to apply the drop of blood.

3. While the monitor is doing its thing, get your drop of blood ready by inserting a fresh needle into the stylus, activating the mechanism that pops the needle into the pad of your finger, and squeezing to draw out a large drop of blood (the monitor will tell you if you have placed too small a drop on the test

strip). Change the finger you use each time you test so they don't get sore.

4. Put the drop on the test strip and let the monitor do the rest. In forty-five to sixty seconds (you can watch the readout display count down), the machine will beep and you have your result. Write the number in your booklet.

5. Clean off your finger, take the needle out of the stylus and the strip out of the monitor, discard them safely in a place where children and pets can't get at them, and you're done. The whole thing takes two to three minutes.

In the beginning, if you feel nervous about doing this yourself, or if you're not sure you're doing it correctly (you probably are if you are following the manufacturer's directions step-by-step), ask a friend or family member to walk you through it the first time or two. You can take the monitor to your physician or nurse practitioner to teach you how to use it, but you'll be charged for an office visit.

Even though you may feel slightly intimidated at first, a SBGM is one of the simplest devices you will ever use. It's no more complicated than setting a digital alarm clock, and it's a thousand times easier than programming your VCR!

When to Test

The short answer is: Test when your doctor tells you to. The longer answer is a little more complex and gives you some leeway to use your own judgment. Here's an example: one day, a few months after I was diagnosed with diabetes, I felt awful. It was nothing I could put my finger on and nothing hurt. I just felt as if I wanted to get under the covers and not come out for a few days. I knew my blood glucose was way up, and when I tested, I was right. It was way over two hundred.

Instead of falling into a panic and calling my doctor, I made myself go out for my three-mile walk. I didn't want to, and I wasn't sure I could manage the whole distance, but I decided to go as far as I could. It was a beautiful fall day: cold enough for a thick jacket and gloves. I started slowly and gradually increased my speed until I was pacing along with a nice spring in my step. I waved to the people raking leaves and stopped to pet a few of the dogs and cats I've gotten to know (I walk the same route every day so my mind is free to think about things other than where I'm going). I finished the three miles, and by the time I got home, I felt fine. In fact, I felt great. Again, I knew my blood glucose was much lower so I tested it and again I was right. It had dropped about fifty points.

The exercise was responsible for part of the rapid and significant drop (see chapter 4 for more about the effects of exercise on blood glucose), but other factors also were at work. The walk both energized and relaxed me, so I was in a much happier and calmer state of mind when I got home. Although you won't find this in any medical text, the glorious weather probably relieved some of the stress I was feeling. And I gave myself a good "talking to" when I was outdoors: I told myself not to be afraid, that whatever was wrong was fixable, that my doctor was only a phone call away, that I had done really well so far with my diabetes, that I had lost a lot of the weight I wanted to, and that I was generally an okay person. Moreover, I was not about to drop dead on the spot. In short, I relieved my stress, which has a significant effect on blood glucose. There is more about the effects of stress in chapter 8.

So, when do *you* need to test your blood? In the beginning, because your glucose levels can vary so much and your diabetes is not yet under good control, you will need to do it several times a day: before you eat breakfast in the morning and then after lunch and supper. People who take insulin usually are told to test at least four times a day.

When you have your disease under fairly good control, you can decrease the number of tests to once a day or even every other day, but always on the advice of your doctor. Monitor your glucose level at the same time every day for about a week, so that whatever fluctuations you find are an accurate representation of the glucose in your bloodstream rather than vagaries of diet or the time relationship of eating to testing. In other words, if one day you test right after you have gotten up in the morning and before breakfast, and the next day you do the test after a heavy meal, you're going to see some pretty wild differences that don't mean what they seem. So test at the same time each day for a week, and then the next week you can monitor at a different time of day every day for a week.

In addition to your regular testing schedule, there are some special times when you should keep more frequent track of your blood glucose:

- If you think you are having an attack of hypoglycemia (low blood glucose). If you look pale and feel shaky, sweaty, weak, dizzy, and hungry, or if your heart speeds up and your lips feel numb and tingly, you may be having a hypoglycemic episode. Test your blood glucose right away, and if it's below 70 mg/dl, you need treatment (see chapter 9).
- If you are ill, even with just a cold, test your blood two or three times a day because glucose can increase significantly (a condition known as hyperglycemia) during physical illness. If it goes above 240 mg/dl and stays there for two consecutive tests, call your doctor.
- If you are taking a short-term medication for something other than diabetes.
- If you have changed the times at which you take your diabetes medication or if you make major changes in your lifestyle: increasing or decreasing your amount of physical exercise, working a different shift, traveling through a few time zones, or going through a particularly stressful event.
- When you are on vacation or a business trip.

Keeping Records

Writing down your SBGM results each time you do the test gives you an accurate picture of how well your diabetes is controlled. But it does more than that:

- It provides important information about the decisions you make regarding what to eat and how much to exercise.
- It shows you the juxtaposition of whatever medication you are taking with your dietary management and blood glucose levels.
- It shows you immediately when you have to make changes in your diet or lifestyle. For example, if you have had a rough week at work and are very stressed and have not had time to take your usual bike rides, that will probably show up on the monitor, and you will know that you have to make some adjustments.

It's tempting to become disheartened, or even downright panicky, when one or two SBGM results are too high. Let's say you've stuck to your food plan (I hate the word "diet" and will try not to use it often in this book), and you've been walking your two or three miles a day rain or shine, and still your blood glucose is over two hundred twice in a row. Don't worry about it; just keep doing what you're supposed to be doing. Many things can elevate your numbers, even for a few days at a time: you might have a cold or some other little infection you're not aware of, you might not be testing at the same time every day, you might be undergoing severe stress, or you might have forgotten to factor in a medication that you are taking temporarily.

Getting a Grip on Emotions

When my doctor called me that Friday evening to tell me that I had diabetes, I was shocked, because bad news is always a shock. But later, in an effort to be scrupulously honest with myself, I wasn't really surprised. Although I don't know of any relatives who were diabetic, my lifestyle was terrible. When I look back on the way I used to live, it seems as if I did everything possible to bring out whatever tendencies toward diabetes were lurking in my genes.

But all that first evening and most of the next day, I had all the symptoms of emotional shock: I felt disoriented, I had trouble thinking clearly, and I felt as if I had been run over by a truck and was lying helpless in the street. The numbness and sense of physical assault wore off by Saturday night, though. Nature doesn't allow shock to last indefinitely, and I knew I had to start coping with the disease, to accept the diagnosis, and to mobilize my emotional resources.

Besides, I had been invited to a dinner party that evening and had been looking forward to it all week. I told myself that I'd be damned if I'd let a little thing like diabetes prevent me from having a good time. So I set out for my friend's house in a state of false euphoria. I had no idea what Larry was going to serve for dinner, but on the way to his house, I vacillated from resolving to eating everything in sight to eating practically nothing. What really happened was that I proved to myself that I could achieve one of the most important things a diabetic must learn: I could moderate my eating habits.

It wasn't easy—not by a long shot. Larry always serves cheese and crackers with drinks before dinner, and I love cheese. I also enjoy a weak Scotch and water with hors d'oeuvres. So I compromised; I had two small pieces of cheddar on crackers instead of several large slabs of brie on French bread. And I passed up the Scotch in favor of a glass of wine that I knew would accompany dinner.

Dinner wasn't much of a problem because Larry has always been health conscious and doesn't cook with much fat, but he is a great dessert cook. This evening, he had outdone himself with a "killer" chocolate cake. He brought the cake to the table and everyone groaned with delight. The women, as usual, said, "Just a small piece for me," and for once, I added my voice to theirs. Larry didn't listen, of course; he knows me well. A four-inch wedge of cake was placed in front of me, and my mouth began to water.

I was faced with a dilemma: If I refused the cake, people would ask what was wrong, and then I'd have to make a decision about what to say. If I ate the cake, which I dearly wanted to do, I would be hurting myself. So I ate half, licked the last morsel of frosting off the fork and set it neatly on the plate next to the uneaten portion of cake. And there it sat, tempting me like the Sirens of Greek mythology luring sailors to their death on the rocks. Everyone at the table was chatting and drinking coffee, and there I was, unable to think about anything else but that lovely dark confection. I willed myself to keep my hand off the fork, but the self-imposed discipline was taking all my energy and I couldn't force my concentration away from the damn cake.

Suddenly, I had a bright idea. I got up from the table, took the plate of cake into Larry's kitchen, dumped it down the disposal, went back to the dining room, and enjoyed the rest of the evening. Larry looked at me quizzically, and I told him I'd explain later.

What I did that evening was much more than throw out a piece of cake. I took control of a difficult situation. I made a decision to be good to myself, take care of myself, and solve a problem that at first had seemed insurmountable. That was the first step in taking control of my diabetes. I have been in tough spots since then, and I will be again. Sometimes I do give in and finish the entire piece of cake, but more often than not, I say, "No, thank you." I will talk more in chapter 3 about techniques and strategies for controlling what you eat, but suffice it to say here that "control" and "choice" are the operative words.

A man in a support group that I sat in on once said something interesting about the issue of control in diabetes: "If you want to live a long, healthy life, get a chronic disease and take good care of it." He was right. When you learn all the elements of diabetes management, your entire physical well-being will improve and you'll probably end up healthier than most of your nondiabetic acquaintances.

Stress

Having a serious, chronic illness is stressful. There's no way to deny the fact of the stress, but there are ways to cope with and minimize it. First, though, let's look at some of the reasons why many people are so stressed when they hear the diagnosis, as well as some of the factors that affect stress levels.

Many newly diagnosed diabetics know little or nothing about diabetes and therefore suffer from serious free-floating anxiety, which is usually worse than being afraid of something specific. In addition, most of the things they know about diabetes are wrong, and therefore they have to correct myths and unlearn misperceptions. For example, one of the most common incorrect ideas about diabetics is that they can never eat anything with sugar in it. The thought of no more desserts for the rest of your life is indeed pretty stressful. Luckily, it's not true.

Familiarity with health concepts in general and the way the body works in particular seems to affect the amount of stress people have when they get a serious illness. The more you know about human anatomy and physiology (body structures and the way they function), the easier it is to learn about diabetes, and the better you understand the disease, the easier it is to cope with it.

The amount of confidence people have in their ability to solve problems and make life changes affects stress level. If you can say to yourself, "This is pretty serious stuff, but I've dealt with things that are just as bad so I can deal with this, too," you are on your way to significantly lowering your stress level. People who feel unable to overcome every obstacle that life tosses in their paths are going to suffer significantly more stress when they find out they have diabetes. Age also makes a difference. The older one is, usually the easier it is to cope with diabetes, as well as crises and problems of all sorts.

Thinking about a lifetime of unhealthy eating habits is stressful, especially if you've known better for a long time. Discussing these past "sins" with a physician or nurse practitioner is no fun either. In fact, it's downright stressful. However, it may help reduce your stress to realize that there is nothing that can be done about these past mistakes, and that there is a lot that you can do to improve your current and future health.

Some people fear what others will think about them for having diabetes, and fear causes stress. The good news is that this fear is based on a false assumption. Except for your physician, close family (whom you probably want to tell anyway), maybe one or two people at work to come to your aid in the event of hypoglycemia (if you are Type I), and your health insurance company, no one else has to know that you are a diabetic. The disease doesn't show on the outside, and you are under no obligation to explain anything to anyone. Later, when you get used to the idea of having diabetes and are less stressed about being able to take care of yourself, you may want to tell more people, but you never have to.

Anxiety over what the disease will cost—immediately and over a lifetime—can get your adrenaline pumping. We will discuss money matters in chapter 10, but for now, suffice it to say that all supplies, medications, blood tests, and trips to the doctor or nurse practitioner are covered by health insurance or are tax deductible.

You may need help coping with and minimizing stress. This comes from a variety of sources. The first and most important is to acquire accurate and helpful information about what diabetes is, how it affects you specifically, and what you can do to control it. Reading this book and talking to your health care provider are a good start to this solution.

Second, when you feel stressed about your diabetes, remember you are not alone. Of course, you already know that you're not the first person in the world to get diabetes, and you may realize that it is an extremely common disease (there are about fourteen million diabetics in the United States, with 500,000 diagnosed each year), but that probably won't make you feel less alone. Support groups are one answer to the problem (see chapter 7), and talking to close friends and a wider range of family members is another way to let others help alleviate your stress.

It is also stress relieving to rely on your own inner strength. Once you know what you are dealing with, when you learn how to control the "big, bad monster" that has appeared in your life, and you realize that you can do it, it will probably occur to you that this isn't nearly as bad as you thought it would be. On that day, you will breathe a sigh of relief and incorporate the fact of having diabetes into your life as easily as you have incorporated other things that you wish were different: having curly instead of straight hair, not being able to carry a tune when you love to sing, suffering from terrible seasickness so you can't go sailing with your friends, or being violently allergic to cats.

Fear

Uncontrolled diabetes really is something to be scared of. It's a serious, potentially fatal disease. If you don't take care of yourself and learn to control the disease, some pretty awful things can happen.

Driving a car is something to be really scared of. Driving a two-ton machine at seventy miles an hour—only a few feet from other two-ton machines—is a serious, potentially fatal endeavor. If you don't do it with care and learn to control that machine, some pretty awful things can happen. When you're a teenager behind the wheel for the first time and you release the brake and roll out into traffic, you're petrified. There seem to be a thousand things to remember, and it feels like millions of other vehicles are racing toward you, intent on crashing into you—or at least trying to make your life on the road thoroughly miserable.

In reality, there are only a few things to remember about the mechanics of driving: accelerating, braking, steering, and watching what's going on around you. And in reality, there are only two or three cars at any one time that are close enough to ram into you, and most of the time you can control your distance from them. It's the fear that makes you feel out of control and panicky. Diabetes is similar.

In reality, there are only a few things to remember about the mechanics of diabetes control: your blood glucose, the food you eat, and your amount of physical activity. And there are only two or three serious side effects that you have to worry about at any one time, and you almost always have some control over how serious a threat they become.

It's good to recognize that people have realistic fear—it keeps them on their toes and prevents them from doing stupid, dangerous things. It's not good to allow that fear to grow and develop until it paralyzes you and you can't release the brake and roll out into traffic, or you're too scared to test your blood glucose, or you're unable to think clearly about whether to have dessert tonight or save it for Saturday evening when you're out on the town.

Use your fear of diabetes to take control of the disease, but if you find your fear controlling you, call your doctor and ask to be referred to someone to talk it over with (a psychotherapist or a diabetes educator).

Anger

It is entirely normal to be angry, even wildly furious, for a while when you find out you have diabetes. You're right: it isn't fair. You may be angry at practically everyone: your parents for the genetic endowment they gave you—and for getting you into bad eating habits in the first place; your doctor for insisting that you have the blood test and for giving you the bad news; your spouse or partner and children for not having the disease or not reacting to your news in the way you wanted them to; and most of all, yourself.

Your anger may be everywhere. It comes with the fact of having a lifelong illness. The problem is not that the anger exists—it is human to feel angry at something this big and this serious. Rather, the problem is coping with the anger, directing it toward useful channels, and letting it escape in appropriate ways.

Naturally, people are not angry all the time, and the anger at having diabetes will most likely be short lived. But because anger affects all relationships, strategies for channeling it in useful ways should be directed toward preventing the opening of old wounds, narrowing whatever rifts exist among family members and friends and guarding against letting the anger leak out in ways that might be ultimately harmful.

There are a variety of techniques that people have developed to release anger harmlessly: playing high-energy sports; writing down their feelings; going somewhere where no one can hear them scream, shout, curse, and otherwise carry on in what most people would consider an unseemly fashion; and talking out the anger with a professional listener, such as a clergyperson or therapist.

> *Vivian was furious at herself for waiting so long to go to the doctor when she had every symptom in the book. "My sister has diabetes and my mother had it, and I knew what was wrong with me, but I stubbornly refused to get that blood test.*

Then when I finally couldn't postpone it any longer, my glucose was really high."

Why did she wait so long? She didn't want to have to deal with it. She knew that taking care of herself wouldn't be as bad as she thought, because she'd watched her sister do it for a few years, but facing the reality wasn't something she was ready for.

Vivian is in perfect health now. Her hair shines, she has a beautiful figure—not too fat, not too thin—and she has clear skin. She watches her diet like a hawk. Instead of the hamburger, fries, and milkshake she used to get at lunch, now she more often opts for a veggie burger and a diet soda. However, she is not a vegetarian, and still eats meat and desserts as part of her carefully regulated diet.

Vivian got over her anger at herself and learned to accept the reality of diabetes. She controls it with diet and exercise, and she knows more about the physiology and chemistry of the disease than a lot of physicians. She went to diabetes classes and read everything she could get her hands on. That helped a lot in getting over her anger.

Denial

Denial is a powerful emotional tool that often can be used to good advantage. However, when diabetes rears its head, denial is not appropriate. It is tempting, but foolish.

Denying the seriousness, or even the existence, of diabetes is dangerous because it will prevent you from getting the help you need, and it will delay or prevent you from learning to control the disease. The longer you delay getting your blood glucose under control, the more likely you are to suffer serious health effects down the road.

People use a wide variety of denial mechanisms to protect themselves from the reality of diabetes. Some intellectualize the disease and collect vast amounts of medical information on the subject, but they don't do anything practical with it. Intellectualization is a way to deny feelings and manage stress, and can be used positively or negatively. Learning everything that it is possible for a layperson to understand about diabetes and its management is one way to increase control, but the knowledge has to be put to personal use.

Some people turn to religion for strength in the face of what they perceive as an overwhelming disaster. (Diabetes can be a major inconvenience in your life, especially at first, but it is by no means a disaster.) While feeling spiritually supported is comforting and can give you strength, you also need to take care of your own health and reap the benefits of treatments and control techniques researched and developed in medical laboratories.

Still others never accept the diagnosis and trudge from doctor to doctor (or from alternative healer to alternative healer) seeking a quick fix, thus denying themselves the advantage of scientifically accepted treatment and control. If you decide to try alternative health options, do so only in addition to the treatment recommended by your medical doctor.

Finally, there are people who believe that, with all the current medical research on diabetes, a cure is just over the horizon. So they deny the immediacy of their situation and sit back and wait, or they hope that their diabetes will go away by itself if they ignore it, or they believe that it is their doctor's responsibility to take care of them and get their blood glucose levels down to normal. All these assumptions are wrong and dangerous.

Using denial as a psychological technique can have benefits as well as disadvantages. Denying feelings of hopelessness and helplessness can force people back onto the track of practicality and control. It also can lessen the preoccupation with the disease that comes naturally to most diabetics when they are first diagnosed, and it can minimize the fear that so often accompanies all bad news. Denial can be especially useful when its direct result is positive action.

Charles and his buddy Steve used to sit on Charles's front lawn every afternoon after work and well into the evening—in just about any weather—and drink prodigious amounts of beer. (It was only later that Charles stopped denying his alcoholism.) One day, Steve walked over to Charles's house unannounced to borrow a garden tool and found him almost unconscious in his backyard shed. He was pale, sweaty, and almost incoherent. Steve called 911 and sat with him until the medics arrived. Steve had never even known that Charles was diabetic.

Charles survived the episode, but while he was in the hospital, his doctor told him that, had no one found him, he could have gone into a diabetic coma or even died.

Depression

When anger, grief, and denial are directed inward, they can turn into energy-sapping depression. Not only is this not helpful, it can be debilitating. You need all the strength you can muster to make arrangements for your treatment and get control of your diabetes.

True, it is depressing to be sick, but you are not going to be "sick" for long. Here's how one woman described her reaction when she found out the results of her glucose tolerance test (in which a series of blood samples are drawn over a period of a few hours to determine how the body reacts to drinking measured amounts of glucose solution): "Everything but the diabetes just fell away. There was nothing in my life but that awful disease and the fact that I could actually die of it. It was totally consuming."

This is one way that people experience depression, which has a variety of external and internal symptoms: sadness, crying unexpectedly and for no apparent reason, irritability, insomnia, decreased appetite (or compulsive eating), restlessness, boredom, diminished sex drive, lack of interest in appearance and diminished physical energy—sometimes to such an extent that a person ceases to function.

Joyce, a fifty-four-year-old woman, found out she had Type I diabetes. She had a family history of serious illness, as both her grandparents died of heart disease, both her parents now have heart disease, and her father is a diabetic. Joyce had a sort of resigned hopelessness about her health and her life, and she was scared to death all the time. She was a severely depressed woman.

Joyce was also depressed about other aspects of her life: her romantic partner, her job, and her repetitive daily routine. These were problems before she found out she had diabetes, and they will continue to be problems for her as she attempts to improve her health. Because of her lack of energy, caused by the depression, Joyce had a hard time dealing with her diabetes, and every day she put off making changes, she felt more depressed. She has, however, finally begun taking psychotropic medication, and consequently feels more hopeful about the future.

If you feel depressed about your diabetes or other issues in your life, take care of yourself by seeing a therapist and working through your problems. Most people who have recently learned that they have diabetes have a lower grade of depression than Joyce. They may feel mired in gloom for a few weeks, but they soon learn to pull themselves out of it. Here are a few ways to combat such feelings:

- Dress in bright, cheerful clothes. Get dressed every day, even if you don't have to show up for work.
- Have plenty of green plants and fresh flowers around. Tend your garden or start one.
- Engage in a pleasurable activity at least once a day, even if you are especially busy at work. It may be something as simple as sitting in the sun for fifteen minutes and eating an apple, but it has to be something you take pleasure in.
- Exercise every day. A long walk with a dog (yours or a neighbor's) is calming.
- Stay in the light as much as possible, especially in winter. Go outdoors on sunny days and keep your indoor environment well lit.
- Structure your day so you don't have huge blocks of time with nothing to do. Depression characteristically feeds on itself; keeping your mind occupied with external activities prevents you from dwelling on depressing thoughts. If necessary, write your activities down on an hour-by-hour basis so there's always a goal to be accomplished.
- Plan activities in advance—preferably with other people so that you are obligated to do them.
- Don't do things that you know will depress you. For example, if you have heard that a movie is a real tear-jerker, don't see it. If a book you're reading is making you feel terrible, set it aside until you feel better.
- Seek professional help from your medical doctor, a therapist, or a psychiatrist.

3

Food As a Key to Control

The goal in controlling diabetes is to maintain blood glucose levels as close to normal as possible for diabetics: 80–140 mg/dl fasting or 100–180 mg/dl one or two hours after meals. The best way to do this is to eat the healthiest diet you can and lose weight. (Since the vast majority of people with Type II diabetes are overweight, I am making the assumption that you need to shed 30 or 40 pounds.)

You have probably heard all kinds of horrific things about a diabetic diet (for example, no dessert or alcohol for the rest of your life) and how difficult it is to follow. You may believe you practically have to be a chemist to work out all those food exchanges and calorie and carbohydrate calculations. None of this is true.

But wait. Before you run off to scarf down a hot fudge sundae, there are things about what you eat that will have to change. Yes, you are going to have to get your nutritional act together, and yes, you will have to think about what you eat and plan for certain events. But it's not nearly as bad as you think it's going to be.

Scientific thinking about a diabetic diet has changed in recent years. Things used to be very rigid, with instructions to eat a half cup of this and no more than a quarter cup of that, and there were strict exchange groups. And it used to be true that you could never put a drop of sugar in your mouth and that carbohydrates in general were strictly limited.

Things have changed for the better for diabetics. Now, if your blood glucose is in reasonably good control, you can eat a much wider variety of foods. What you really have to watch out for is fat—but everyone should be doing that. The damage that saturated fat does to the body has been so widely publicized that eating a low-fat diet has become the "in" thing to do for many people. You should now be one of them.

> *When Dolores found out she had diabetes, all she could think about was the food part. She'd been on a million diets and always felt deprived. It got so that sometimes she couldn't pay attention at work because huge peanut butter and strawberry jam sandwiches floated across her mind.*
>
> *Because Dolores always treated herself so harshly whenever she went on a diet, they never lasted, and she ended up "falling off the wagon" with a bang: She would buy a whole jar of peanut butter (extra crunchy) and eat most of it at once—without the bread and strawberry jam. Then, of course, she'd feel guilty and terrible about herself, the diet would be "ruined" because of that one slip, and she'd gain back all the weight she had lost.*
>
> *Dolores is now a diabetic, but she still eats peanut butter and jelly sandwiches—her favorite food. She doesn't do it very often, and she plans for them and works them into her diet. While peanut butter is not one of the preferred foods for diabetics, it is important to Dolores to be able to eat it, so she has learned how to control the amount she eats and when she eats it. Her "thing" with peanut butter has helped her to pay attention to and understand her eating patterns and her feelings about food.*

This is the crux of using nutrition to help control your blood glucose level: understand what you are eating, plan what you eat, control the amount, and decide when you are going to eat it. If you can do this, you have gone a long way toward controlling your diabetes.

And while you are thinking seriously about changing and improving your eating habits, you will eventually learn what works best for you. Just as Dolores learned to come to terms with peanut butter, you will learn what you can't live without, what you can eat in moderation, and what really doesn't matter as much as you thought it would.

My thing is ice cream. I used to eat it almost daily. When I was diagnosed with diabetes, I knew I couldn't do that anymore so I made a bargain with myself: My rule is that I can eat as much ice cream as I want once a month. The first time I put the rule into effect, about two months after my diagnosis, I ate an entire quart of chocolate chip at one sitting and got sick. I still have the ice cream rule, but I usually don't eat more than a pint because, odd as it seems to me, I don't want more than a pint. I still love ice cream as much as ever, but too much high-fat food all at once no longer appeals to me (I know about low-fat ice cream, but I don't like the taste).

Eventually, you will find out which foods make your blood glucose go up and which don't affect it as much as you thought they would, and you'll learn how much you can eat at one meal while keeping your blood glucose in control.

Terry was at a week-long conference, during which she shared most of her meals with the same people. After a while, people noticed how little she ate at each meal—about half as much as everyone else. A few were rude enough to comment on the amount of food she ate. At first, she said nothing, but they persisted, so she explained that when she was at home working, she usually ate five or six small meals a day (she didn't say why), and at the conference, where food service was controlled by someone else, she couldn't manage the big portions. She didn't tell them that she had found a grocery store a few miles away, and that she had a stash of health snacks in her hotel room. It was important to Terry that no one at work know of her diabetes, so she managed to explain herself to her colleagues without discussing it.

While you need to do what you have to do to keep your blood glucose in control, you also need to eat the way you like to eat and keep at least some of your lifelong food habits intact.

Several years ago, the U.S. Department of Health and Human Services issued general guidelines for a healthy diet for everyone. It included suggestions to eat a variety of foods; lower dietary fat, particularly saturated fat and cholesterol; increase intake of starch and fiber; avoid too much sugar and sodium (salt), especially in processed foods; and drink alcoholic beverages only in moderation. The agency publicized these recommendations in the form of a food pyramid. Breads, cereals, rice, and pasta form the base of the pyramid (six to eleven servings recommended every day). The next level up is vegetables (two to three servings) and fruits (two to four servings); the second-to-top level includes milk, yogurt, and cheese (two to three servings) and meat, poultry, fish, eggs, dry beans, and nuts (two to three servings). At the top of the pyramid are fats, oils, and sweets (use sparingly). This is how you should be eating.

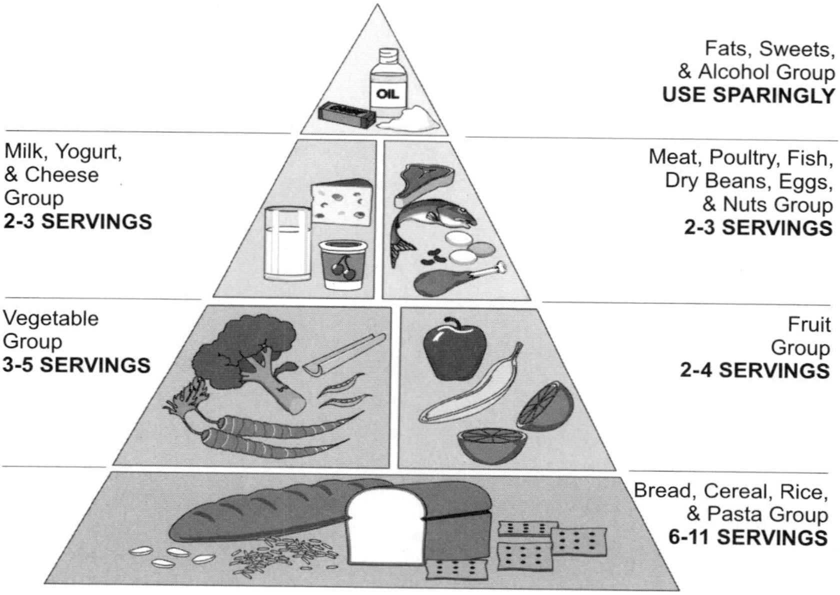

How Nutrients Affect Diabetes and Insulin Production

Food is one of the major things that affects diabetes, and it is a strong factor in preventing complications. All foods are made up of nutrients: carbohydrates, proteins, and fats, as well as vitamins and minerals. Each type of nutrient has it own effect on blood glucose.

The effect of eating these nutrients depends on the total amount in your diet and on your own individual metabolism. The longer you monitor your blood glucose and the better you learn to correlate the results with what you have eaten prior to the test, the better you will come to know the short-term and long-term effects of carbohydrates and sugar on your blood glucose.

Carbohydrates

Carbohydrates, which are composed of a variety of sugar molecules, are known as sugars and starches and are the body's major source of energy. In addition, carbohydrates build and repair body tissues and regulate most body functions. Without them, you would die. There are two major types: simple and complex. Simple carbohydrates are sugars such as lactose (found in milk), glucose, fructose (found in fruits and vegetables), and sucrose (cane or beet sugar). Anything that tastes sweet contains one or more types of sugar.

Complex carbohydrates, so named because they are chemically more complicated than simple sugars, are found in starches such as bread, pasta, and rice, and some vegetables such as beans, potatoes, and corn. Fiber is a complex carbohydrate as well.

Both simple and complex carbohydrates are broken down by the body into glucose, which is the substance you measure when you test your blood. Simple and complex carbohydrates are broken down at the same rate, and they both provide four calories per gram. However, different foods produce differing amounts of glucose. Two major factors influence how high your blood glucose will go after eating: the amount of carbohydrate per serving and the speed with which the carbohydrate is converted into glucose. The latter depends on how big the servings of food are, whether it is cooked (digested faster than raw), and how much liquid the food contains (the more liquid, the faster it is digested). In addition, if you eat carbohydrates in combination with other nutrients, the carbohydrates are digested more slowly. This is why it is not a good idea to eat a candy bar as an emergency treatment for hypoglycemia; the fat from chocolate and fiber from nuts slow down the digestion process.

Carbohydrates and sugars elevate blood glucose faster than any other nutrient because carbohydrates are digested rapidly and become glucose quickly. If you don't have enough insulin in your bloodstream to counteract a sugar surge, your blood glucose could rise abnormally. However, this does not mean that you can never eat sugar. First of all, it would be impossible because sugar is an inherent part of so many foods, and second, eating some carbohydrate and sugar is an essential part of a healthy diet.

Ever since the American Diabetes Association relaxed its food guidelines for diabetics, carbohydrate counting has become popular. The ADA noted that there was no scientific evidence that supported the restriction of foods containing sugar. That is, the effect of carbohydrates is the same on blood glucose regardless of the source. So ten grams of carbohydrate from spaghetti will act the same in your body as ten grams of carbohydrate from a piece of cake. This is good news indeed.

However, it doesn't mean that you can go out and stuff yourself with sugar. You still have to count total carbohydrates, but it makes meal planning a good deal easier, and it allows for an occasional gooey dessert.

Your dietician or other health care provider will determine, based on your blood glucose level, medication, and exercise level, how many grams of carbohydrates you can eat in a day. You decide in what form you will consume that total—within reason. For example, you should not use up your entire carbohydrate allotment for one meal in the form of sugar, but if you are in a situation where you want to join others in eating a significant dessert (a birthday party or other social gathering), you won't fall into an immediate diabetic coma, nor do you need to feel as if you have totally messed up your food plan. In such an instance, however, if you are a Type I diabetic, check your blood sugar immediately afterward.

There are other reasons for controlling the amount of sugary food you eat. Most of the time, they are lacking in other nutrients and provide what has become known as "empty calories." Portion size of high-sugar food is also smaller than low-sugar foods. For instance, you can eat an entire cup of sugar-free yogurt for the same carbohydrate "price" of a third of a cup of regular fruited yogurt.

Fiber

Fiber is a carbohydrate found in vegetables, grains, fruits, and nuts. It is the part of the plant that cannot be digested. Since it is not absorbed, it does not provide calories, but because it is so bulky, it helps make you feel full. Obviously then, fiber is a good thing to eat when you're trying to lose weight. The only problem is that it's not particularly emotionally satisfying. (No one's mother ever said, "I'll give you a nice piece of broccoli if you behave yourself.")

Water-insoluble fiber, such as wheat bran, helps the digestive tract by keeping waste products moving through the intestines, thus preventing constipation. Water-soluble fiber (oat bran, wheat germ, legumes) slows the passage of food from the stomach into the intestines, and it may help lower cholesterol.

Proteins

Protein is the basic building material of human life; it is used to create and repair tissue. Much important body tissue is composed of protein: muscles, bones, organs, and chemicals such as hormones and neurotransmitters. Protein also can provide energy in the absence of carbohydrates. For example, if you were to lose so much weight that you used up all your fat reserves and were not taking in enough carbohydrates to provide energy, your body would start breaking down muscles and other tissues and use the protein they contain to keep you going. This is one of the things that happens to people who suffer from anorexia nervosa.

Twenty-two amino acids, combining with one another in an almost infinite number of sequences, form the basis of protein. Your body manufactures only thirteen of the twenty-two; therefore the other nine must come from the food you eat. Protein is found in both plant (grains, legumes, nuts) and animal (meat, poultry, dairy products, fish) sources. Protein provides four calories per gram.

Fat and Cholesterol

Dolores had a harder time controlling her intake of fat than of sugar. This is probably true of many of us because fat, even more than sugar, is what makes things taste good. You hardly ever hear people say that they would rather eat low-fat cheese or salad dressing than the regular kind. Fat molecules carry the flavor of foods, and when their globular little selves are removed from ice cream or cheese or cookies, much of the flavor is removed also. Beware of packaged products touted as "low fat." The manufacturers usually add extra sugar to compensate for the absence of fat. Later I will explain how to determine if this is what has happened by reading the nutritional labels on food packages.

Most people know there is a difference between saturated and unsaturated fat. The former is generally solid at room temperature and comes from animal products (milk, eggs, meat), except for palm oil and coconut oil, which come from plants but are saturated. Unsaturated fat is a vegetable product (olive oil, corn oil, safflower oil) and is liquid at room temperature.

Cholesterol, which is not a fat but works in conjunction with fat in your body, is a waxy substance that gets into your bloodstream via two major routes: it is manufactured normally by your liver and intestines, or it enters through the food you eat. Fatty red meat, whole-milk dairy products, and eggs are examples of foods high in cholesterol.

Cholesterol is deposited on the walls of your arteries, where it builds up over the years, gradually narrowing the lumen (inside passage) of these blood vessels, limiting the amount of blood that can get through. Eventually, the artery may become completely clogged, resulting in a heart attack or stroke.

Your body manufactures two types of cholesterol: high-density lipoprotein (HDL) and low-density lipoprotein (LDL). HDL is often called "good" cholesterol because one of its actions is to remove cholesterol from the arteries and carry it back to the liver where it is reprocessed and sent on its way to be eliminated. LDL is deposited into the arteries, and is the kind of cholesterol you want to minimize in your diet.

Fats work in concert with cholesterol in the following ways: Saturated fat raises the level of LDL, which increases your chances of clogged arteries. Unsaturated fat is believed to lower LDL levels and may even help raise HDL. For this reason, you should make an effort to eat more polyunsaturated than saturated fats. Try not to eat more than 300 mg of cholesterol each day.

There are a number of reasons why you need to limit your intake of fat and cholesterol. For one, fat is a significant factor in the development of cardiovascular disease (heart attack and stroke), and as a diabetic you have an increased risk of these health problems. To reduce the risk, reduce your fat intake.

Eating a high-fat diet is also one of the things that makes you overweight. One of the best ways to lose weight is to cut way down on fat in your diet. Each gram of fat you eat has twice the calories of each gram of carbohydrate or protein. If you were to eliminate fat completely from your diet (which is not healthy to do), you would automatically cut your caloric intake in half.

Finally, muscle tissue has more insulin receptor sites than your body chemistry is able to accommodate. Therefore, when you lose body fat, which lies close to the muscle, you eliminate one of the factors that may be interfering with insulin receptor sites.

One way to reduce fat intake is to keep track of the grams you eat. This is easier than you may think and you don't have to be a mathematician to do it. All you do is keep a daily running total, using a chart showing the grams of fat in various foods. Then you choose foods that add up to your daily total. It's exactly like calorie counting—only with fat grams.

How do you find out how much fat is in various foods? You read the label of prepared foods and you buy a book that has a list of the fat content of other foods. Any big bookstore will have a wide variety of them, or you can write to the U.S. Government Printing Office for a copy of "Nutritive Value of Foods," a free pamphlet (see Resources for address).

Vitamins and Minerals

Vitamins and minerals are an integral part of the nutritive value of food, and if you eat a balanced diet, you do not need to take additional vitamins in the form of pills. Taking megavitamins (huge doses of selected vitamins) has been touted as a cure-all for a number of ailments, but megavitamins can be extremely harmful, and in some cases, fatal. The same holds true for minerals such as calcium, potassium, iron, and zinc. Having diabetes does not increase your need for vitamins and minerals.

Making Choices about Food

Just about everyone has formed some kind of emotional relationship with food. It starts when they are children and is a direct result of the way they were introduced to food, the use their parents made of food in their upbringing, and the types of issues that their immediate families had about food.

Dolores grew up in a family where everything was fried, which explains why she has a thing for fatty foods. She explained that as she grew up, her taste in food became more sophisticated, and she threw away her deep fryer. But she never got over her craving for foods that contain a lot of fat and oil, hence her deep attachment to peanut butter.

With some people, their love is for sugar. Babies naturally love a sweet taste, and many American parents added sugar to their infants' water bottles to calm them or make them stop crying. As these babies were weaned, sweet foods were substituted for sugar water as a reward or a bribe.

People eat for a variety of reasons, many of them having nothing to do with hunger. They eat as a social function, because they're bored, depressed, or elated, or as a way to nurture themselves. Whatever the reason, the choices you make reflect a long-ingrained need for certain types of food.

Weight Loss

Most people with Type II diabetes have been on more than one diet in the past (Type I people tend to be naturally thin). Those diets have been more or less successful—for a time. But the weight almost always comes back, usually in greater measure than what was lost in the first place, so that over the years the pounds escalate—slowly but steadily.

Many also have tried every fad and crash diet that has come along and have been able to stick to those for less time than a "regular" diet. Some people have even been desperate enough to try surgery: removal of a large part of the small intestine where nutrients are absorbed, insertion of a balloon in the stomach to create a feeling of fullness, or gastric stapling to decrease the size of the stomach. These procedures work for a time, but they, too, ultimately fail and weight goes back up.

Crash diets are useless for the most part, but for diabetics, they can be especially dangerous. Most of them do not constitute what could even remotely be thought of as a balanced diet and are thus lacking in specific nutrients (and overloaded with others). If you are taking insulin or oral hypoglycemic agents, a nutritional imbalance could lead to serious hypoglycemia or hyperglycemia.

There is, alas, only one way to lose weight and keep it off: eat less and exercise more. The details of a weight loss diet are a bit more complex, but in the end, those are the essentials. It's a matter of burning off more calories than you take in, so that your body will have to use stored fat as a source of energy rather than rely on what you feed it.

Reducing calories can slow down metabolism, the rate at which you burn calories. Therefore, it is especially important to increase your physical activity when you begin your weight reduction program, because exercise increases metabolism. It's a two-part process, both of which are equally important.

Maintaining a reasonably normal weight is especially important for diabetics for a number of reasons:

- Excess weight places an added strain on the cardiac, vascular, and respiratory systems, which predispose one to cardiovascular pulmonary diseases, of which diabetics are at higher risk than nondiabetics. One important way to minimize risk is to lose weight.
- In Type II diabetes, being overweight interferes with the body's ability to use insulin. Losing weight alone, that is, without taking medication, often results in a significant drop in blood glucose. Even a loss of ten to twenty pounds, or 10 percent of your body weight, will show up as a pleasant surprise on your blood glucose monitor—as well as on your bathroom scale.
- Weight loss affects the amount of insulin or oral hypoglycemic agent that a diabetic requires. In some cases, losing sufficient weight means that you don't need to take medication at all.

Your nutritionist or other health care practitioner will tell you how many calories you should eat in a day, and you probably already know how to count calories. There are, however, some tricks you can play on yourself to lower your caloric intake, while barely noticing the "loss" and without feeling as though you're eating nothing but "rabbit food." By the way, have you ever noticed that most rabbits are quite plump?

- Trim all visible fat off meat and poultry. You'll retain the taste of the meat but greatly reduce the calories it contains.
- If you don't want to drink skim milk because it's too thin or looks strange in your coffee, use 1% or 2% milk (and other dairy products). The flavor will come through the way you like it, but you will cut your fat calories by 50 to 75 percent. Use skim milk in recipes; you won't be able to tell the difference.
- Give up real sour cream. Try substituting yogurt, or mix it in equal parts with low-fat sour cream. It tastes almost like the real thing.
- Remove the skin from poultry before you eat it and never fry it. Consider Southern fried chicken a relic of the past—or a semiannual treat.

- Give up butter, lard, bacon fat, and shortening; cook with liquid oils. You may find that your food actually tastes better, because it won't be overwhelmed by the taste of the grease.
- When baking, use three-quarters the amount of sugar called for in the recipe. If it tastes fine (and it probably will), try cutting the sugar content down to two-thirds.
- Skim the fat off soups and stews. If you can, make them the day before, refrigerate overnight and then peel off the solidified fat. These kinds of foods often taste better when allowed to rest for a day anyway.
- Try not to eat eggs as a food (no more cheese omelets as a midnight snack). Think of them only as an ingredient in recipes.
- Avoid sweet alcoholic beverages such as liqueurs, cordials, and sweet wines. If you must have a drink after dinner (more about alcohol later in the chapter), take a small glass of dry wine or nonmalt liquor.
- Drink only diet sodas and use artificial sweeteners in your coffee and tea.
- Don't eat sugar-coated cereal or chew sugared gum.
- Eat dried fruits only in moderation, and use the unsweetened variety of foods such as jelly, jam, condensed milk, canned fruit, syrups and the like.
- Think very carefully and plan ahead for desserts.
- Eat smaller portions, and stop eating when you're full. Don't worry about insulting your hostess if you don't finish everything on your plate, and don't allow yourself to be talked into second helpings if you don't want them or shouldn't have them. Resign your membership in the "clean plate club."
- Think about where you are and what you are doing when you eat high-fat, high-sugar foods (usually snacks). Do you grab a bag of salted peanuts when you settle in front of the TV? Do you stop at a Dairy Queen on the way home from work? Do you always help yourself from the office doughnut supply? Try to break these negative eating habits.
- If you know you are eating as a reaction to emotional stress, use other ways to deal with the stress, such as exercise, taking a bath, or talking to a friend.

- Stay out of fast-food restaurants unless you promise yourself that you'll stick to the salad bar or grilled chicken.

You may already know about the above hints and techniques, and there are many more you could add to this list. But none of them is helpful unless you have already made a commitment to yourself to lose weight. No one can talk you into it, and you lose weight for no one but yourself. No matter how long and hard you have been encouraged (even nagged) by family and friends, your weight reduction program won't be successful until you are committed.

Diabetes can be the impetus that finally does the trick. It often works that way with other diseases. A man who keels over from a heart attack spends some of his time in the cardiac care unit evaluating his lifestyle (and his high-fat diet) and resolves to mend his ways. A woman whose blood pressure goes through the roof and results in a stroke learns to throw away her salt shaker and read food labels as she is learning to navigate her house with a cane or walker.

In many ways, it's a matter of what you value and what's important to you. No one can guarantee your safety on the highway if you obey the rules, don't speed, and keep your distance from other cars, but your chances of reaching your destination safely are increased if you drive safely. By the same token, there's no saying for certain that you will suffer the dire consequences of diabetes if you don't lose weight and get control of your blood glucose, but the risk will be greatly increased. It's your choice.

Making a Food Plan

Without thinking about it, you already have a food plan. Everyone does. It may not be as healthy as it could be, but it's a plan. Most people who shop and cook for their families have a general idea of what they're going to prepare for the next few days or for the week. You at least know you're going to eat several meals a day, and you spend at least some time thinking about what you're going to have for your next meal. Most adults know how to cook, if even in a very basic way. If you don't know how, it's a life skill worth learning—and a whole lot less expensive than eating in restaurants all the time.

There are a number of elements to consider in making a diabetic food plan, all of them with a great deal of flexibility built in.

First, you need to take a realistic look at your lifestyle. Do you travel a lot for business? Are you a workaholic who seldom eats at home? Are you a grazer who rarely sits down to a proper meal? Second, you will need to correlate what you eat with the medications you are taking. For instance, when do they reach their peak action, and how often do you take the medication? Third, do you have any other medical conditions that affect your diet? And finally, what food restrictions do you live with, for example, are you a vegetarian? Do you keep kosher?

When you create a food plan for yourself, don't think of it as a diet (even if it really is). That's a depressing word that can conjure up images of hunger, deprivation, and isolation. Try to think of it instead as simply one of the several lifestyle adjustments you are making to control your diabetes.

The American Diabetes Association Guidelines and exchange lists are located in the appendix. You should become familiar with them as you create meal plans, and you might even want to photocopy those pages and carry them in your purse or briefcase for when you go grocery shopping or eat in a restaurant.

Shopping for Groceries

An important part of planning meals is going to the grocery store and buying the ingredients for what you've planned to eat. "Come on," you may be thinking, "I've been doing the family food shopping for longer than I want to think about. I know the store by heart and there's nothing you can tell me about how to shop."

This may be true, but have you ever turned the package over and read a food label? Or if you have, have you ever gone beyond the calorie count? Most people don't, but now that you have diabetes, it's a good idea to learn how. Luckily for all of us, in 1994, the Food and Drug Administration redesigned and standardized the labels so that each manufacturer of prepared food must use the same format. The new law applies to all foods manufactured in the United States and to those imported for sale here. Every label must show how much total carbohydrate (including dietary fiber and sugars), sodium, cholesterol, and fat a product contains, and it must list the amount of saturated fat, protein, minerals, Vitamins A and C, and—perhaps most important—the total calories and calories from fat.

Let's go through the major elements of a food label:

NUTRITION FACTS

Serving Size One Hot Dog (45 g)
Servings Per Container 10

Amount Per Serving

Calories 45 **Calories from Fat** 15

	% Daily Value*
Total Fat 1.5 g	**2%**
Saturated Fat 1 g	**5%**
Cholesterol 15 mg	**5%**
Sodium 430 mg	**18%**
Total Carbohydrate 2 g	**1%**
Dietary Fiber 0 g	**0%**
Sugars 2 g	
Protein 5 g	

Vitamin A 0%	*	Vitamin C 8%
Calcium 0%	*	Iron 2%

* Percent daily values are based on a 2,000 calorie diet. Your daily values may be higher or lower depending on your caloric needs:

	Calories:	2,000	2,500
Total Fat	Less than	65 g	80 g
Sat Fat	Less than	20 g	25 g
Cholesterol	Less than	300 mg	300 mg
Sodium	Less than	2,400 mg	2,400 mg
Total Carbohydrate		300 g	375 g
Dietary Fiber		25 g	30 g

Calories per gram:
Fat 9 * Carbohydrate 4 * Protein 4

- **Content versus percent of daily value.** The top part of the label lists nutrients as a percentage of what an average person requires based on a two-thousand calorie diet, and the bottom part of the label lists the actual amount of a nutrient in that particular package. For diabetics, the top is a general guide, and the bottom is an essential part of your food plan.
- **Serving size.** I have always thought that food manufacturers must believe that they are packaging their products for a flock of birds because the serving size is always so small. Who eats a half cup of chocolate pudding? You might—when you look at the number of calories in a serving size that looks like only a thimbleful in your dish. You might also decide it's not worth your while to spend that many calories on such a little bit of prepared food. You might also realize that it's too hard for you to eat only a half cup, and you might be tempted to end up finishing the entire container. Whatever your eating habits and food preferences, be sure you note the serving size and have a good idea of what half a cup looks like on a plate—or you could actually measure it. The amount of nutrients described on the label refer to each serving, not to the entire container.
- **Total carbohydrates.** This should be a major focus of your attention. Remember that it is the total amount of carbohydrates

you consume, rather than individual kinds of sugar and starch, that affects your blood glucose.

- **Types of fat.** Choose foods that have the lowest percentage and total amount of saturated fat.
- **Ingredients.** The ingredients of the food in a package are listed in descending order by weight. The first four or five items are usually the major ingredients, and the rest are flavorings and chemicals used as preservatives. Therefore, it's important when buying prepared foods such as frozen dinners to see what they actually contain so you can match them to your meal plan. In addition, the picture on most packages provides a fairly accurate idea of what you will find inside, although it won't taste nearly as good as it looks.

As you get into the habit of reading labels, you'll come across some terms that you've never heard before or that you don't know the meaning of. Many items on the supermarket shelf have the words "healthy" or "natural," most of which have no regulatory meaning. The federal government (the Department of Agriculture regulates labels on meat and poultry products and the Food and Drug Administration regulates seafood, processed food, dairy products, and produce) controls what manufacturers are allowed to claim about their products. Here's what the label terms mean:

- **Low fat:** no more than 3 grams of fat per serving for individual foods, and no more than 30 percent of calories from fat for complete meals
- **Low in saturated fat:** no more than 1 g of saturated fat per serving, and no more than 15 percent of total calories from saturated fat
- **Fat free:** less than 0.5 g of fat per serving
- **Low sodium:** 140 mg or less per serving
- **Sodium free:** less than 5 mg of sodium per serving
- **Light (Lite):** one-third fewer calories or 50 percent less fat per serving
- **Low cholesterol:** no more than 20 mg of cholesterol and 2 g or less of saturated fat per serving
- **Cholesterol free:** less than 2 mg of cholesterol and 2 g or less of saturated fat per serving

- **Reduced/less:** contains 25 percent or less of a nutrient than a comparable food
- **Low calorie:** no more than 40 calories per serving
- **Sugar free:** less than 0.5 gram of sugar per serving
- **Dietetic:** does not necessarily mean the item is good for you; it means that something has been changed or replaced in the food: salt, sugar, total fat, or cholesterol
- **Natural:** in regard to meat and poultry it means that no chemical preservatives or hormones have been added; for other foods this has no regulatory meaning

You also need to know how to figure the percentage of calories from fat. Here you need to use a little arithmetic, but it's not hard—and it *is* important. Because each gram of fat contains 9 calories, all you do is multiply the grams of fat per serving (it's right on the label) by 9 and then divide this number by the total number of calories in each serving. To convert to a percentage, multiply by 100.

For example, a food that contains 4 grams of fat and 100 calories per serving is calculated as follows:

4 grams of fat x 9 = 36 fat calories

36 ÷ 100 (calories per serving) = 0.36

0.36 x 100 = 36% of the calories comes from fat

Eating Away from Home

In general, you eat away from home the same way you do at home except that you have somewhat less control over what you choose. Unless you're in the hospital (where there will be a professional dietician available to you) or in prison, eating out should pose no great problem. Most restaurants have such a varied menu that you will have no trouble finding things that fit into your food plan. Not only that, but many have what they call "dieter's sections" on the menu or there are items highlighted as being "heart healthy" or "lean cuisine." And you can always ask the waiter how the food is prepared. Don't be embarrassed; people ask this all the time.

There are some specialized restaurants that might give you pause, but there are ways to deal with them, too.

- *Fast-food joints.* The best thing is not to go into them in the first place, but if you absolutely can't help it (you're with a group of co-workers and you're the only one who votes no to fast food, or you're on an interstate and you're starving and there's no place else to eat), choose the salad bar with low-fat dressing or grilled or roasted chicken (not fried). As a last resort, eat a hamburger, but hold the cheese and the mayonnaise.
- *Italian restaurants.* Choose a tomato-based sauce on your pasta instead of one made with cream, and eat chicken or fish prepared relatively plainly. Try to stay away from lasagna and veal or eggplant parmigiana; they're loaded with high-fat cheese.
- *Delicatessens.* Most delis now have a wide variety of salads (avoid salad with a high-fat mayonnaise dressing), but if you want a sandwich, stick to lean roast beef or poultry. Traditional deli meats (corned beef, pastrami, tongue, brisket of beef) are among the highest-fat proteins. Never eat chopped liver, and when you're having a bagel with cream cheese and lox, ask for the low-fat variety or use only half a portion of regular cream cheese.
- *Chinese restaurants.* Watch out for food that's deep fried: anything that's described on the menu as "crispy" is usually rolled in a coating of some sort and dropped into hot fat. If you're eating soup, stay away from crunchy Chinese noodles; they're prepared the same way.

Other ways you can be good to yourself in restaurants include staying away from the bread and butter before your appetizer or entree is served. If you're really hungry, ask the waiter for a small plate of raw vegetables such as carrots, radishes, or celery, or order a salad—that usually shows up quickly. Ask for low-fat dressings or request that it be served in a small dish on the side. If the waiter balks at this, consider this attitude when it comes time to leave a tip. Don't forget that you are the paying customer, and the restaurant needs to please you, not the other way around.

When you're invited to someone's home for dinner, things become a little more difficult because you usually have no choice in the food that is offered to you. There are still things you can do to maintain control, however, and even if you can't, don't forget that it's only one meal.

If the home you are invited to belongs to a close friend, they may already know that you are a diabetic and serve something appropriate to your needs. If you can't say something beforehand about food preferences, it's usually better not to mention that you have diabetes. This can throw people into a panic about what to feed you, and they'll watch you anxiously all evening to see if you're about to collapse onto their dining room table. It'll make everyone uncomfortable. Rather, eat a smaller amount of food and if you feel the need to explain, try something like, "I'm trying to shed a few pounds, so please don't be offended if I eat lightly." This is something everyone can relate to, it's a polite warning, and no one gets put on the defensive.

If you have chosen to say nothing in advance, and most people prefer not to, you can still do fine at someone else's table. Here are some ways to stay in control:

- Have only one drink before dinner—heavily diluted with water or diet mixer. Keep your wine consumption during dinner down to one glass or less (more about alcohol and diabetes later in this chapter).
- Look over the hors d'oeuvres choices and choose the least caloric and fat filled. Take the raw vegetables (and don't dip them into anything) instead of the cheese, or if there is only cheese and crackers, choose the hardest cheese (which contains the least fat) and eat it without a cracker. Stay away from things like cocktail weenies rolled around pastry, salted nuts, and crunchy snacks poured right out of a bag. The good thing about this part of the meal is that people are concentrating on each other, and no one notices what kind of snacks you are or are not popping into your mouth.
- At the dinner table, eat what fits into your diet, and don't eat what you don't want to. Your obligation is to yourself, not to your hosts. You can always say you're allergic to something if there's a comment.
- You can eat part of what you're served: Cut the steak in half; peel the skin off the chicken if it's fried or greasy looking; scrape off cream sauce before you eat what's under it. If anyone says anything, say that the food was delicious but you're stuffed and can't eat another bite. This comment could also work to get you out of eating dessert if you want to pass.
- If you're invited to a cookout or barbecue, try to choose a meat you can eat without a bun. Choose the coleslaw, three-bean salad, or rice or pasta salad, and leave the mayonnaise-soaked potato salad alone. Fill up on watermelon and fruit and have

only a small cookie or piece of brownie for dessert. Drink light beer, diet soda, or unsweetened iced tea (carry your own packets of artificial sweetener in case there is none available).

Cooking for the Family

The support of a loving family is one of the most important elements of successfully controlling diabetes, especially in terms of food preparation. Whoever cooks for a family with a diabetic person should prepare meals as if everyone is a diabetic. This sounds harsher than it is; your family will end up eating healthier because, as you now know, a diabetic diet is really not much different from a generally healthy diet. The portions can vary among family members, and there's no reason why other members of the family can't eat other things for snacks and meals that they prepare for themselves or eat away from home (such as lunch.) If your teenage son polishes off half a bag of Oreos when he comes home from school, it doesn't matter as long as you're not joining him. Everyone else can eat potato chips while you're munching unbuttered popcorn during a televised football game. This way, they eat healthier for more meals and can still make separate food choices, and you can have the peace of mind that your family is supporting you while still having times to make their own food choices based on their health needs.

Living and Cooking Alone

The good thing about living alone and cooking for yourself most of the time is that you have total control over what you cook and eat. The bad thing is that people who live alone tend to become sloppy in their eating habits, at least some of the time. Some single people, especially those who are recently widowed, separated, or divorced, dread the dinner hour because it's a time that potential loneliness can rear its head.

Preparing your own meals and eating dinner alone most of the time does not have to be an unpleasant experience. In fact, many people prefer it. There are ways to make the experience enjoyable—and to avoid doing it all the time. You do not have to live on commercial frozen dinners reheated in the microwave, slapped-together bologna sandwiches, or take-out Chinese food. Neither must you eat in restaurants every day.

Treat yourself well. Set aside a time with "real" food that you've cooked yourself; eat at the kitchen or dining table set with nice dishes and a flower or candle. This is a psychological and nutritional necessity. In addition, it creates a pleasant interlude between the day's and evening's activities. Many people like to read or watch the news while they eat. Others enjoy listening to a favorite recording. Still others like to do nothing but concentrate on the food. If you've put effort into cooking something delicious (or even if you've stopped at the deli on the way home for a gourmet salad), take the time to enjoy it. If the phone rings while you're eating, say you'll call back later or let the machine take the call.

Prepare meals that are interesting and that conform to your food plan but that don't require you to spend hours in the kitchen every evening. For instance, cook a pot of stew or hearty soup one weeknight or Saturday afternoon, divide it into single portions and freeze them. Buy food that lends itself to single portions instead of large lumps that you'll tire of before you finish: a few brussels sprouts instead of a whole cabbage, broccoli stalks instead of a whole cauliflower, cut-up chicken parts instead of an entire roaster, and shrimp or salmon steaks instead of a roast. Keep plenty of pasta and rice in the house to combine with vegetables or chicken. Or keep it simple: A grilled eggplant sandwich, raw zucchini and carrot sticks, and an apple takes about ten minutes to prepare but is as nutritionally sound as a full meal that took hours.

Vegetarianism

If you are a vegetarian, you may well be on your way to eating a diet that has great potential benefit for cardiovascular health. In general, a vegetarian diet is higher in carbohydrates than one containing meat, which means that your blood glucose levels immediately after eating may be higher than usual. To counteract this effect, try increasing the fiber content of your meals, which causes glucose to be absorbed more slowly, or try eating smaller, more frequent meals.

Making Choices about Alcohol

It is a common belief that diabetics are not allowed to drink any alcohol at all. This is not true, but you should drink it in moderation because alcohol has an immediate effect on blood glucose, it's high in calories, and it tends to stimulate your appetite.

Twelve ounces of light beer, 8 oz. of regular beer, 4 oz. of wine, and 1.5 oz. of hard liquor each contain one hundred calories. If you take insulin, don't try to compensate for the calories in alcohol by cutting back on food intake. You need all the nutrients in your meal plan. If you're not on insulin, do deny yourself some carbohydrate food in order to make up for the alcohol calories.

You should not have more than two alcohol equivalents a day, and you should separate the two drinks by at least two hours. An alcohol equivalent is either a 4 oz. glass of wine, a 12 oz. light beer, or a mixed drink containing 1.5 oz. of hard liquor diluted with diet mixer. This means two drinks on any one day. In other words, if you go for a week or two, or even a month, without having a drink, you cannot "make up" for not drinking on those days by having more than two drinks when next you drink.

Alcohol's effect on blood glucose is immediate and significant. You know how fast it gets into your bloodstream because you can feel how fast it reaches your brain. In fact, unlike food, alcohol is absorbed directly from the stomach into the bloodstream and is carried to the liver where it is metabolized (broken down, absorbed by cells, and then excreted). While the liver is working on the alcohol, it "forgets" to release glucose so your blood glucose levels can sink to dangerous lows in a very short time. The reaction can last for a very long time—up to thirty-six hours, well after you have recovered from the other effects of drinking.

In addition to the fact that alcohol is fattening and plays tricks on your liver, it also can worsen diabetic neuropathy, and if you are taking the oral hypoglycemic Diabinese, you may experience harmless but frightening facial flushing and you may get a bad headache.

Try to reserve alcohol consumption for special occasions instead of a regular part of your life. You don't need wine with dinner every evening, and if you regularly stop off at a bar on the way home from work, you ought to look at why you need to drink as a celebration for leaving work or as a shield to face going home. But if you don't want to give up the ritual or the camaraderie, every now and then ask for a nonalcoholic beer or a half-strength mixed drink.

At parties and receptions where there is a bartender, ask for a half-strength drink (and watch the bartender as the alcohol is poured), and on the second go-round, have your glass filled only with mixer. That way you can have a glass of wine with dinner.

When you don't want to drink or when you have had your quota for the day, simply say, "No, thank you." Say it with a smile and don't offer any explanations if you choose not to. This is what recovering alcoholics do, and most people are getting used to accepting that some friends and colleagues choose not to drink.

Don't drink on an empty stomach, as the alcohol will reach your bloodstream even faster with no food to absorb at least part of it. If you are going to a restaurant where a drink is the first thing served, eat a snack before you leave the house or office, or if you are having an appetizer, ask that yours be served with your drink. At dinner at someone else's house, eat a few appetizers before you have your drink. If there aren't appetizers, and you don't know the hosts well enough to go into the kitchen to get a little snack, don't have an alcoholic drink until dinner.

Problem Drinking

If, when your diabetes was diagnosed, you had an alcohol problem or if you are an outright alcoholic, you must stop drinking altogether; if you haven't already, call up your local chapter of Alcoholics Anonymous (AA) and attend a meeting. AA is probably the most effective way to help people stop drinking, but it is not the only one. Decide how you want to stop drinking and then do it.

4

Physical Activity

Many people hate the word "exercise." It conjures up images of sweat-soaked young women—with great figures, skin-tight leotards, and pert little ponytails—prancing around a mirrored room to loud music. Or it brings to mind muscle-bound studs lifting hundreds of pounds of weight—sweaty and grunting. You may think of neighbors you see pounding the pavement as they run their six miles before breakfast, looking grim and determined.

If you share this aversion to exercise, you may think you'll never be able to do something like that. Just thinking about it may be so exhausting that you collapse onto the couch and continue your imitation of a potato. Well, you don't have to go to these extremes. Only a small minority of Americans are fanatic exercisers (but we all have the shoes for it!).

But you are going to get off the couch and start moving.

Exercise means physical activity, and the more physical you are, the more calories you burn—and the better you are at keeping your blood glucose in control. But exercise is not only jogging or playing tennis or doing push-ups. It's cleaning the house, raking leaves, mowing the lawn, pulling weeds, walking to work, maintaining your sailboat, bicycling to the grocery store.

Every time you move a muscle (even changing positions in bed at night), your body uses energy. Energy is calories. The more muscles you move and the longer you move them, the more energy your body requires, and the more calories you burn.

Exercise recommendations for diabetics used to be fairly rigid: thirty to forty minutes of moderate exercise three or four times a week. However, new medical evidence shows that physical activity can be just as beneficial if it is mild to moderate but done for shorter periods of time every day of the week. This is good news because one of the major excuses people use for not exercising is lack of time.

However, this doesn't mean that you should not do moderate or intense exercise for longer periods of time as well as shorter stints of physical activity. In fact, the more you exercise (short of hurting yourself or running yourself into the ground from exhaustion), the better off you will be.

Vivian sees exercise as her medication and controls her Type II diabetes with a food plan and exercise alone. She never goes more than two days without her "medicine."

Vivian varies her types of exercise because she gets bored doing the same thing every day. Two or three days a week, she goes to an aerobics class with two women from her office, and other days she lifts weights, walks in a park that has many trails so she can vary her route, uses a treadmill in her basement, and works out with Jane Fonda and Richard Simmons tapes.

Vivian does many kinds of physical activity cheerfully. When she got diabetes, she paid more attention to what she was doing and how often; she wants to see how long she can control her diabetes without having to take drugs. So far, so good. She has had diabetes for eight years. She looks good, feels great, and keeps her blood glucose on an even keel.

Types of Physical Activity

Aerobic Exercise

Aerobic exercise conditions the heart, lungs, and blood vessels by increasing the body's ability to use oxygen and thus minimizing the risk of heart attack, stroke, and other cardiovascular diseases. Aerobic exercise is perfect for diabetics. It is done continuously (without stopping), rhythmically (muscles contract and relax in a regular pattern), in intervals (varying the pace of the activity during the continuous exercise session—fast and slow walking or jogging and walking, for instance), progressively (increasing in difficulty), and for endurance.

Running and walking are the two best aerobic exercises for most people. If you are over forty, you should stick to walking unless you are an experienced runner. Walking provides all the advantages of aerobic exercise, it is free (except for the price of good shoes and socks), everyone can do it, you don't have to go anywhere specific to do it, and you can do it any time.

Walking is good for relaxing, controlling blood glucose, lowering blood pressure, and getting the circulation going (great for your feet). Aerobic exercise also has been known to lower blood lipid (fat) levels, help with weight loss, decrease stress, increase muscle tone and strength, increase the feeling of helping oneself, and lower the risk of osteoporosis.

Excellent aerobic exercises include: jumping rope (for younger people who don't have foot neuropathy); taking aerobics classes (done with an experienced instructor); rebounding on a trampoline; riding a stationary or real bicycle; using a skiing or rowing machine; and practicing tai chi, a Chinese system which, in its 108 moves, involves every part of the body.

Anaerobic Exercise

Anaerobic exercise is usually very intense and uses energy stored in the muscles. Examples are weight lifting and calisthenics. They are not particularly effective in improving cardiovascular conditioning. Calisthenics develop and improve range of motion in joints and muscles. These include bending and stretching, which are recommended as part of warm up and cool down during aerobic exercise. Diabetics will benefit more from aerobic than anaerobic exercise, but the latter is also good for you.

Intensity of Activity

Common sense tells you that there are various levels of exercise intensity. Taking a walk around the block is not the same as jogging five miles, and hiking through the woods for two or three miles on a level path is not the same as climbing a mountain. Exercise specialists divide intensity levels as follows:

- Moderate activity of short duration—walking a mile or bicycling for less than thirty minutes

- Moderate activity of intermediate duration—tennis, swimming, jogging, leisurely bicycling, gardening, golfing, or vacuuming for one hour
- Intense activity of long duration—football, hockey, racquetball, strenuous bicycling, shoveling heavy snow, skiing, or hiking for two hours or more

Approximate Number of Calories Burned in a Half Hour

Exercise	Calories Burned
Sitting	40
Sleeping	50
Driving a car	50
Walking 2 mph	110
Bowling	125
Housework	140
Horseback riding (trotting)	175
Square dancing	175
Swimming leisurely	200
Bicycling leisurely	200
Tennis (doubles), weeding, raking	200
Walking 4 mph	225
Playing golf, mowing the lawn	225
Ice skating	235
Cycling 5.5 mph	250
Scrubbing floors	270
Tennis (singles), digging, hoeing	270
Skiing 10 mph	300
Squash and handball	300
Jogging 5.5 mph	320
Jogging 7 mph	350
Cycling 13 mph	500

If you are taking insulin and you plan to exercise strenuously and/or for long periods of time, you need to consult your physician or a sports medicine specialist about how to correlate food intake and insulin injections with your exercise program.

Health Benefits of Physical Activity

In addition to its calorie-burning advantages, regular exercise is particularly important for diabetics because it helps lower blood glucose, and it has been known to help lower levels of LDL cholesterol in the blood and may even increase HDL cholesterol.

Blood Glucose

Muscles use two main types of fuel for energy: glucose and fatty acids. Exercise works in the following way: during the first few minutes of activity, muscles use their own stored sugar. As the muscles begin to relax and contract, the body uses sugar stored in the liver, which is transported through the bloodstream to the muscles. After about thirty or forty minutes, the body begins to burn its own fat in the form of fatty acid.

Insulin plays a role in physical activity because it enables the body to use glucose for energy. It and other hormones tell the liver to produce more or less glucose and fatty acids, which get burned off by the muscles in the form of energy. In addition, cells become more receptive to insulin. This is one of the reasons why overweight Type II diabetics who begin to exercise and lose weight often can get along without taking oral hypoglycemic agents. Some even find that all or most of the symptoms of diabetes disappear.

Stress

After you have been exercising for a while, you'll notice that you feel better all over. Part of this is due to the fact that you're losing weight and your blood glucose is in better control, but that's not the whole story. Exercise is known to be a highly effective stress reducer. There are a number of reasons for this. First, when you exercise hard or play a competitive sport, you concentrate on what you are doing—on getting the ball over the net in precisely the spot you aim for, assessing your opponent's vulnerabilities, or deciding which garden plants will look better in another spot—and then digging them up and putting them there. This tends to drive all other thoughts from your mind and you stop worrying about the fight you had with your spouse or partner or the work that's piled up on your desk. You take a little mental vacation.

Exercise also releases a hormone called norepinephrine (also called endorphin), which creates a feeling of calm and well-being. The sensation is sometimes called a "runner's high," but norepinephrine is released with any kind of exercise, and it often lasts three or four hours.

There are many psychological benefits to exercise. People who walk the same route all the time at a steady pace often find themselves falling into a relaxing meditative state. If you do group sports or go to a health club or gym, you are likely to meet new people, some of whom might turn into friends. You also lose the guilt that was always nagging at the back of your mind if you were a couch potato. Getting rid of guilt gets rid of a great deal of stress—and it feels great.

Effect of Exercise on Insulin Production

As you begin to plan your exercise program, you should know how physical activity affects insulin production and blood glucose levels. If there is not enough insulin circulating in the bloodstream, glucose cannot get into the cells to provide them with sufficient energy; therefore, it accumulates in the bloodstream. The end result is that the muscles don't get the glucose they need, and your blood glucose climbs higher and higher. In addition, if you exercise often when your blood glucose is too high, you run the risk of ketoacidosis, which can be life-threatening.

If you have too much circulating insulin, the liver mistakenly senses that there is sufficient glucose available for the muscles so it slows its production of the sugar. At the same time, the muscles are using all or most of the available glucose, which makes your blood glucose level drop. This is not good either.

It is important to prevent yourself from falling into a state of hyperglycemia or hypoglycemia while exercising; there are many precautions you can take. Always test your blood glucose immediately before and after exercising. If it is above 240, test your ketones before you begin. Ketones are substances the body produces when it starts to burn fatty acids, and you should not exercise until the problem has been corrected. If your blood glucose is between 240 and 300 but you test negative for ketones and you are a Type I diabetic, it's okay to exercise; a blood glucose above 300 means you should stay put until you can lower it. Type II diabetics should not exercise with a blood glucose of 400 or more.

Getting Started on a Physical Activity Program

One of the worst things you can do to your yourself and your diabetes is to transform yourself from a couch potato into an exercise nut overnight. Most Type II diabetics probably wouldn't do that because they wouldn't be overweight in the first place if they weren't such sluggards (and research has shown that they might not have gotten diabetes if they had been exercising regularly all their lives). But some people demonstrate a rather turbulent reaction to the diagnosis. They want to turn over a new leaf, jump onto the healthy living bandwagon, forswear all sugar and fat, and immediately join a health club.

This new lifestyle usually lasts a very short time because it is too dramatic a change and is difficult to sustain. Try not to do this. It's exhausting and hard on your body and soul. Rather, ease into an increase of physical activity. First, get a physical examination and make sure that you are well enough to become physically fit. If you have had diabetes for more than twenty years, a physical examination is crucial because some exercise may be detrimental. For example, some forms of diabetic eye disease can worsen as a result of constant impact, and if you have heart disease, there are certain exercises you should avoid. More about this in the section "Special Considerations for Diabetics" later in the chapter.

Next, make certain your diabetes is in reasonable control. If your blood glucose fluctuates wildly or if you have a tendency toward ketoacidosis (a buildup of ketones in the blood), get those problems solved before you begin to exercise. Also, think of ways you can incorporate increased activity into your lifestyle without calling it exercise, for example, park in a far corner of the supermarket lot (walking to and from and around the store could add up to a whole mile), get off the bus a few stops early and walk to your destination, climb two or three flights of stairs instead of using the elevator, clean your own house instead of having someone else do it, put the TV remote control in a drawer and haul yourself out of the easy chair to change channels, walk to the grocery store, and buy less food and shop more often.

Change the way you do certain things in order to increase physical activity, for example, stop driving everywhere and start using your legs or bicycle, don't sit for more than an hour at a time, go to other people's offices instead of asking them to come to yours (it'll make them feel more important, especially if you're their boss). Make exercise part of your daily routine. If you think of it as something you just do every day, like shaving, brushing your teeth, or taking time to read the daily paper, you won't have to think about it, and you'll be less likely to moan and groan before gearing yourself up to do it.

Choose Your Physical Activities Carefully

Do activities you like, or at least the ones you hate the least, while getting the most benefit from them. The best type of exercise for a diabetic is one that uses large amounts of energy over a relatively long period of time, what was described above as moderate activity of intermediate duration: tennis, swimming, jogging, leisurely bicycling, gardening, golfing, or vacuuming for one hour. (Okay, so you may not like vacuuming, but you have to do it anyway so you might as well count it as exercise—because it is.)

Other excellent activities include dancing, rowing, fencing, handball, racquetball, digging in the garden, and lawn mowing with a hand mower (if you have a huge yard, trade in your riding mower for a power machine that you walk behind). If you like to engage in exercise with other people, try volleyball, ice or field hockey, soccer, lacrosse, or basketball. Stop-and-go activities such as bowling, golfing with a cart, baseball, and some kinds of calisthenics use only short bursts of energy and are thus less appropriate (although certainly not harmful) for diabetics.

It is best to get some physical activity every day, but if you can't, every other day or four or five times a week is fine. What you should not do is stop and start an exercise program, that is, get out there every day for a month or so and then slack off for a month. Physical activity should be a consistent part of your life.

You also need to think about when you exercise. Naturally, you can't interrupt an important business meeting, no matter how bored you are, to say, "Sorry folks, I'm going swimming at the 'Y' now." But you can incorporate an exercise program into your schedule so it provides the most benefit. For example, the optimum time for physical activity is about an hour after meals when your blood sugar is at its highest. This is easy to accomplish on weekends, but during the week, you have to make a conscious effort. Try eating lunch while you are working and then using your allotted lunch time to take a walk or go to the gym or swimming pool. You probably won't be the only one in your office who does this.

More and more people work at home, which gives much more flexibility about when they exercise. I'm a writer and often work on deadline so self-discipline in my work is important. Therefore, I get up, go into my office, finish the work I have to do for that day, and "treat" myself to a three-mile walk in my neighborhood.

Tips to Increase Physical Activity

Set realistic goals for yourself. It's unrealistic to believe you will lose twenty-five pounds the first month of your diabetic food plan, and just as unrealistic to believe that you will run five miles a day, every day, for the rest of your life. Consider your age, general physical condition, and weight and then make a plan and stick to it. Do not consider the amount of time you have in which to engage in physical activity because you are going to make time for it. You might get away with "I just haven't had the time" as an excuse to your boss for being late with a project, but you can't get away with it when your own health is at stake.

If you decide that you are going to walk a half hour or two miles five days a week, choose a route in the neighborhood where you live or work, and scout out a pleasant hiking trail for an alternative to your usual route. Choose a time that's most convenient for you (it doesn't have to be the same time every day) and do it. Just as you will not let yourself be talked into eating what you choose not to eat, don't let yourself be talked out of sticking to your exercise program ("I'd love to go to a movie, but I have to finish up my work and then take my walk. I could meet you at . . .").

Some people like to exercise with another person or in a group. This is one way to maintain your physical fitness regimen because if you have paid for an aerobics class, you're less likely to skip it, and if you make a date to play tennis or handball during lunch or right after work, you won't want to be rude or disappoint your partner.

If you get bored doing the same kind of exercise every day, don't. There's no reason why you can't vary your physical activity (the jocks call it cross training) by walking twice a week, bicycling with a club every other Saturday, and swimming at your health club on Mondays and Thursdays—or any combination of activities, in any order, that pleases you.

Consider your exercise program an absolute obligation to yourself. It is as important to controlling your diabetes as following your food plan, taking your insulin or oral hypoglycemics, and having your eyes checked every year. Be good to yourself.

Don't forget to reward yourself every now and then for sticking to your exercise program. Get a professional massage, buy a new outfit, soak in a hot tub—again, whatever pleases you. And don't forget to always wear shoes that are in good condition. Check the heels and soles of all your shoes regularly, especially the ones you use for exercise, to see that they are not worn down. If they are, have them repaired or buy new ones. Proper shoes are important to everyone but especially diabetics because they protect the feet, which are particularly affected by peripheral neuropathy.

Safety Factors

As has already been mentioned, be safe and get a physical examination before embarking on a physical activity program. You may be healthy as a horse, but do it anyway and tell your physician the kind of exercise you're planning to do. There may be a more appropriate activity suggested than the one you have in mind.

Monitor Blood Glucose

Monitor blood glucose frequently: three or four times a day during the first month that you are exercising (more often if you are Type I), especially as you progress through the beginning stages to the full program. You should do this for two major reasons: First, you need to be certain that your blood glucose is within the safety range described above, and second, you will gradually learn how your body, especially your blood glucose level, responds to your increased activity. Some people say they can actually feel their glucose level dropping while they're exercising, and when they come home to use their monitor, they're correct. But you should never depend on guesses about what your blood glucose is. The only way to know for certain is to actually prick your finger and test it.

If you are a Type I diabetic, you should not exercise if your blood glucose is less than 100 mg/dl. Have a snack and wait for it to rise. By the same token, if your blood glucose is over 250, test your urine for ketones. If the test is positive, you don't have enough insulin. Take an injection and wait until your ketone level is at trace or normal before you begin.

If you are exercising vigorously or for a long time, you should probably check your blood glucose during the middle of your workout. Bring a high carbohydrate, low-fat snack with you if there are none available in the place where you are exercising.

Adjust Food to Physical Activity

When you exercise, your muscles require more sugar for energy than when you are resting. Therefore, your blood glucose can fall rapidly, and you must be able to maintain a sufficiently high level while you are exercising. In other words, you have to balance the sugar you need for energy, the sugar available from food, and the action pattern of insulin or oral hypoglycemic agent. Over time, you will learn how to balance these three factors without thinking too much about it, but in the beginning, you will need to pay careful attention to your body's energy requirements.

The first rule is to never exercise on an empty stomach. The best time is about an hour after eating, but you won't always be able to manage that. Therefore, the chart "Exercise, Blood Glucose, and Food" will provide a general guideline of what to eat before exercising.

Exercise, Blood Glucose, and Food

Exercise	Blood Glucose	Food
Short duration/ moderate intensity	Less than 100	1 bread, 1 fruit, 1 meat
	100–180	1 bread or fruit
	180 or more	no snack
Intermediate duration/ moderate intensity	Less than 100	1 bread, 1 fruit, 1 meat
	100–180	1 bread, 1 meat
	180–240	1 bread or 1 fruit
	240 or more	no snack
Long duration, high intensity	Consult your physician to check on possibly decreasing insulin and what to eat; test blood glucose every hour	

Adjust Medication to Physical Activity

In addition to using food as a means to control blood glucose during exercise, you may be able to accomplish the same thing by adjusting your insulin or oral hypoglycemic agents. However, do not do this without consulting your physician. Medication changes will depend on the amount of exercise, its intensity and duration, and the type of medication you take.

Exercise-Induced Hypoglycemia

It's pretty embarrassing to pass out in front of a gym full of people, or to keel over in a faint while you're out gardening. It's also dangerous to let yourself go into a state of hypoglycemia while you are exercising. Here are ways to avoid it:

- Exercise after eating when your blood glucose is highest.
- Don't exercise while your insulin is peaking because exercise increases blood flow, which makes insulin work faster.
- Learn the way you respond to exercise, that is, the way your blood glucose fluctuates, and plan your exercise accordingly.
- Have a snack during or after strenuous exercise if you need to.

Use Common Sense

You have great intentions: you're going to shed all that extra weight and get your body toned up so that you'll feel good and look good. Fine, but use some common sense.

- Consider the way you feel. If you are ill or really don't feel well, don't exercise that day. I will discuss this is in more detail later, but for now, suffice it to say that physical illness can wreak havoc on your blood glucose level, so don't compound the problem by exercising in the face of the flu or a cold—or something worse.
- Consider the weather. Dress appropriately. Don't go walking or jogging if there's a solid sheet of ice on the pavement. If it's too hot outside, wait until the cool of the evening, or go for your bike ride early in the morning. If the outdoors won't work, find a mall or a gym with a track and walk or run inside.
- Carry identification with your name, address, and phone number, as well as that of your physician.
- Carry a piece of fruit or some crackers in case your blood glucose dips precipitously.
- If you suddenly don't feel well, or if you get dizzy or begin to sweat more than is warranted by the activity and weather, stop. Go home (ask for a ride or call a taxi if you feel too ill to walk or drive), check your blood glucose, and do whatever is necessary to bring it back to normal. If you can't get it there within a reasonable time, call your physician.
- Warm up and cool down. If you walk, start out slowly and gradually work up to speed. If you run or jog, do warm-up stretching exercises. Take the last block or two of your walk or run, or the last few minutes of the activity, at a much slower speed.
- Dress appropriately. Wear a sweatsuit only when you are warming up or cooling down (and outdoors in cold weather), but take it off when you are exercising. *Never* wear rubberized clothes that are designed to make you sweat more to lose "water weight." You could sweat yourself right into a state of serious dehydration.
- Drink plenty of water when you finish exercising, and on hot days carry a water bottle with you. This is particularly neces-

sary in summer when you have been sweating profusely, but even if it's cold outside you need to drink plenty of water to avoid dehydration.

- If you travel to a high-altitude location, reduce your exercise level because there is less available oxygen.
- Never drink alcoholic beverages before you exercise.
- Exercise regularly, not in spurts. Do some kind of physical activity at least four days a week, preferably five, and follow that schedule every week. Don't exercise every day for a month and then sack out for two weeks. You'll have trouble getting back into it, and you won't be giving your muscles, lungs, and cardiovascular system the most benefit.

Special Considerations for Diabetics

Foot Neuropathy

If you have a great deal of trouble feeling your feet, it may be unsafe for you to do weight-bearing exercises (walking, running, aerobics). Even if your neuropathy is minor or intermittent, you need to check your feet for injuries each time after you exercise and wear the most comfortable shoes you can find (don't buy a pair that has to be broken in, they need to feel good right away), and you may want to buy special exercise socks that have extra padding where your feet get the most pressure.

Advancing Age

In general, if you behave sensibly and follow all the guidelines outlined above, people of any age can exercise. However, if you are over fifty, it is essential that you tell your physician that you plan to begin an exercise program. You might need a stress test first. The test will determine your exercise safety level and will act as a baseline for cardiovascular function in the event of future problems.

Older people should probably vary the type of exercises they do. As you age, your muscles lose their elasticity, and it takes longer to repair themselves in the event of even slight damage. Except for walking, it's best not to do the same kind of exercise more than two days in a row. Some people change off every day.

People Who Take Insulin

After you become accustomed to matching the amount of exercise to the amount of insulin you take, follow the same regimen all the time. However, there will be times when you increase your amount of exercise (a pick-up softball game after work or an impromptu volleyball contest on the beach), so you must either take less insulin or eat more food.

Most Type I diabetics would rather eat a little extra than take another shot, and most physicians don't want you to mess around with the dose of insulin that works well. However, you have to do something to compensate for the increased physical activity so make sure you keep a snack kit handy or stop at a convenience store on the way.

Do not inject insulin into the part of the body that's going to be especially heavily exercised. For instance, if you're the pitcher, use your leg instead of your arm. If you're going on a marathon bicycle trip, use your arm for the shot. The reason for this is that insulin absorption is speeded up at the site of injection when intense muscular activity takes place there. Overly fast absorption could bring on an unwanted reaction.

Eye Problems

Choose activities that do not bounce your body, which may harm small blood vessels in the eyes. Try walking instead of running, swimming instead of jumping rope, and low impact instead of high impact aerobics. Avoid weight training and other exercises that put strain on the eyes.

Heart or Kidney Problems

Under a physician's supervision, choose aerobic exercise that will increase cardiovascular fitness. Always do the exercises at no more than moderate intensity and make certain you have adequate warm-up and cool-down periods.

Check your blood pressure regularly, and make certain you increase your fluid intake if you have kidney problems. This will compensate for the fluid you lose by sweating and will prevent dehydration.

5

Medications

Oral Hypoglycemic Agents

Oral hypoglycemic agents are often called glucose-lowering agents, and some people refer to them simply as diabetes pills. They are used only in Type II diabetes in conjunction with a meal plan and exercise program for people whose blood glucose cannot be controlled with diet and exercise alone. It may be that when you lose sufficient weight and get your diabetes in control, you will no longer need to take pills. This is often the case. An oral hypoglycemic agent is not insulin.

How Oral Hypoglycemics Work

Oral hypoglycemic agents work only if pancreatic cells are capable of producing insulin, as they stimulate the pancreas to release more insulin and use it more effectively. This is why Type I diabetics cannot take oral hypoglycemic agents: If no insulin is produced, there is nothing for the oral hypoglycemics to work on. Oral hypoglycemics are most likely to be effective in people who develop diabetes after age forty and who have had it for less than ten years.

Some Type II diabetics have more insulin than they need, but their cells are unable to process it effectively. Oral hypoglycemic agents help control diabetes on both fronts: insulin production and management. They also increase cells' sensitivity to insulin (or decrease their resistance); the result is that the pancreas produces less insulin, but the body uses it more efficiently. In addition, oral hypoglycemics prevent the release of too much glucose stored in liver and prevent it from flooding into the bloodstream in amounts greater than the available insulin can handle. Some types help the body absorb glucose from food more slowly in order to give the insulin you are producing time to act.

Who Takes Diabetes Pills

Your physician will prescribe oral hypoglycemic agents for four general reasons: if diet alone does not keep blood glucose at or near normal levels, if you are getting insufficient exercise to control your blood glucose, if your blood glucose stays too high even in the face of appropriate diet and exercise, or if your blood glucose creeps up slowly over many years.

Again, your physician will tell you how and when to take your medication, but in general they should be taken before or with meals, and skipped doses should not be made up. If you accidentally forget to take your pill, just wait until your next regularly scheduled dose.

Types of Oral Hypoglycemic Agents

Sulfonylureas

Sulfonylureas stimulate the pancreas to produce more insulin. Within this class of drugs, there are two types: those that have been available for many years, known as "first generation," and those that have been developed fairly recently, called "second generation."

First generation sulfonylureas include Orinase (tolbutamide), Tolinase (tolazamide), and Diabinese (chlorpropamide). Second generation drugs are Glucotrol (glipizide), Glucotrol XL (glipizide GITS), Micronase and Dymelor (acetazolamide), and Glynase PresTabs and Diabeta (glybenclamide).

These drugs are generally taken before meals, and occasionally they may be given along with insulin or in combination with other oral hypoglycemic agents. Type I diabetics should not take sulfonylureas, nor should pregnant women or people with serious heart, kidney, or liver disease. Those who are allergic to other sulfa drugs should steer clear of sulfonylureas.

Biguanides

Biguanides, which have just recently been approved for use in the United States, decrease release of glucose stored in the liver and increase cells' sensitivity to insulin. They can be effective for people who had been taking sulfonylureas for long periods of time and for whom those drugs no longer work. Sometimes they are used in combination with sulfonylureas.

Biguanides include Rezulin (troglitazone), a new drug that treats insulin resistance, and Glucophage (metformin). Rezulin acts at insulin's two major target organs, the liver and skeletal muscles, by targeting a specific receptor. In muscles, Rezulin improves glucose use by stimulating muscle tissue to absorb it. In the liver, the drug helps decrease glucose production. Because Rezulin allows the body's own insulin to work more effectively, blood glucose levels fall over a period of weeks. Then, as insulin resistance is lessened and glucose levels fall, elevated insulin levels in the plasma (the fluid in which blood cells float) also fall. Thus, Rezulin treats the primary cause of Type II diabetes, and some scientists believe that the drug may actually preserve pancreatic function and significantly delay or even prevent the need for insulin. So far, Rezulin has no significant side effects.

Glucophage helps body cells use glucose more efficiently without increasing insulin production. It has few side effects. Some people find that they lose weight on Glucophage, and the drug does not cause hypoglycemia, which can be a side effect of sulfonylureas and of insulin. It also has been known to lower levels of blood lipids, an added bonus.

Alpha-Glucosidase Inhibitors

The newest oral hypoglycemic agent is Precose (acarbose), which slows digestion of carbohydrates. Delaying absorption helps slow the rise in blood glucose that occurs immediately after eating (postprandial hyperglycemia), which in turn improves long-term blood glucose control. Precose belongs to a class of drugs called alpha-glucosidase inhibitors that block the action of an enzyme that breaks down carbohydrates into glucose in the small intestine. Therefore, less glucose enters the bloodstream, which gives the pancreas more time to pump out sufficient insulin. Some people experience gas and diarrhea when taking Precose, but this disappears shortly. Precose is sometimes given to Type I diabetics.

Common Oral Hypoglycemic Agents

Drug	Frequency	Duration of Action
Orinase	2–3 times a day	6–12 hours
Diabinese	1 time a day	Up to 60 hours
Tolinase	1–2 times a day	12–24 hours
Dymelor	1–2 times a day	12–24 hours
Glucotrol	1–2 times a day	12–24 hours
Glucotrol XL	Variable	Up to 24 hours
Diabeta	1–2 times a day	16–24 hours
Micronase	1–2 times a day	16–24 hours
Glynase PresTabs	Variable	12–24 hours
Amaryl	1 time a day	Up to 24 hours
Glucophage	2–3 times a day	4–8 hours
Precose	3 times a day (with meals)	4 hours
Rezulin	2–3 times a day	4–8 hours

General Precautions and Side Effects

Any drug that is potent enough to have an action on the body is potent enough to have a reaction. In general, oral hypoglycemic agents are very safe, but you should be certain to ask your physician about possible side effects. They should be given to you when a drug is first prescribed, but some physicians are not as conscientious about this as they should be. Many side effects are only temporary and disappear as soon as your body gets used to the drug. Sometimes they can be made to disappear by reducing the dosage or switching to another drug of the same class.

Many pharmacies now routinely give you a sheet of paper with each filled prescription that lists side effects and the conditions under which you should not take a drug (called contraindications). It is usually tucked into the bag in which the pill bottle is packed. Read it carefully. If you are not given this information, ask for it.

One thing you must be especially careful of is the reaction that an oral hypoglycemic agent might have with a drug you are taking for another medical condition, even a temporary one like antibiotics to treat an infection. Some medications cause diabetes pills to lose part of their effectiveness (for example, some diuretics, corticosteroids, birth control pills, and estrogen supplements). Be absolutely certain that you tell both your physician and your pharmacist about every drug you take.

Each drug has its own particular side effects, but in general, these are the things you should watch out for:

- **Low blood sugar.** If your diabetes medication stimulates your pancreas to produce too much insulin, your blood glucose level may drop and you can become hypoglycemic. Symptoms include shakiness, hunger, nervousness, sweating, dizziness, weakness, irritability, and heart pounding. Test your blood glucose right away; if it's below 60 mg/dl and doesn't rise to normal within a half hour, call your physician.
- **Weight loss.** Weight loss in combination with oral hypoglycemic agents may result in low blood sugar. If you were considerably overweight when you started taking the pills but have been steadily dropping pounds, you may notice yourself becoming hypoglycemic. Tell your physician; this may signal a need to lower the dose or discontinue the medication altogether.
- **Upset stomach.** You may have intermittent stomach and intestinal upsets and loss of appetite. They usually disappear in time.
- **Skin problems.** Skin rashes and itching generally disappear, but if they do not, your physician can change your medications. When alcohol is drunk with Diabinese, sometimes one sees facial flushing. The reaction is startling but harmless and disappears quickly.

Oral hypoglycemic agents have been known to fail. It is not clear why this happens, but if they don't work for you, it is not your fault. There are two types of pill failure that happen occasionally. Primary failure means they never work at all, even when they are first prescribed. Possibly, you were misdiagnosed and really have a very late onset Type I diabetes. Secondary failure occurs after the oral hypoglycemic agents have worked for a while, often years. It happens gradually, perhaps because the body is producing less insulin, or it may be triggered by an unrelated infection, stress, or disease.

The failure might also be due to "user error," that is, when a person with diabetes abandons their food and exercise plan in the mistaken belief that the pills will do everything. You still have to follow your prescribed food regimen, and you still have to exercise. Diabetes is a disease for life, and controlling it is a lifelong project.

If secondary failure occurs, your physician may switch you to a different type of oral hypoglycemic agent or you may have to temporarily be maintained on insulin.

Insulin

Diabetics use either animal or synthetic human insulin. The latter is manufactured by means of genetic engineering, and its biomolecular structure is identical to the insulin produced by the human body. Insulin must be injected; if it were taken orally, it would be destroyed by the juices and enzymes in the digestive tract.

It is measured differently from most of the drugs you are familiar with: in units, abbreviated U. It is manufactured in two strengths in the United States: U-100 and U-500. The former, which most people use, means there are one hundred units of insulin in one cubic centimeter (abbreviated cc) of liquid. You must use a special insulin syringe, which is calibrated in units, to draw the proper dosage out of the vial. An ordinary syringe used to give regular injections will not work.

Types of Insulin

There are three basic types of insulin: short-acting (also called regular or "R"), intermediate-acting (NPH or Lente), and long-acting (Ultralente). They vary according to how quickly the insulin starts to work (onset), when it reaches the acme of its activity (peak), and how long it continues to work (duration).

In the early years of insulin therapy, there was only short-acting insulin and diabetics had to take several injections a day. Now that there are three major types, you have the ability to create a better imitation of the way insulin is normally secreted by the pancreas in reaction to blood glucose levels.

It is, of course, more difficult for you to match injected insulin with your body's needs than it is for a normal pancreas to do it because, in addition to the type of insulin used, a variety of factors affect its absorption and the speed at which it begins to work: the injection site, the depth of the injection, your body temperature (which is actually the temperature of the circulating blood), the time you eat, and the amount and type of food you have eaten.

Short-acting insulin begins working within thirty to sixty minutes of injection, reaches its peak two to four hours after injection, and is completely dissipated within six to eight hours. If you took only short-acting insulin, you would need an injection about every six hours—day and night. Regular insulin is a clear solution.

A relatively new product, very short-acting insulin called Humalog (lysine-proline analog or lispro), works within five minutes after injection, which means that diabetics can more precisely match mealtime and amount of food eaten to insulin injections. Moreover, because lispro insulin spends so little time in the body (about two hours), there is less risk of hypoglycemia.

Because it is so short acting, lispro will not overlap with the next dose; therefore it must be taken in combination with a longer acting insulin in order to provide coverage between meals and at night. The usual regimen is two injections a day of intermediate-acting or long-acting insulin and three injections a day, with meals, of lispro. Lispro is one of a group of "designer" insulins (more will come on the market shortly), which means that they are the result of computer manipulated amino acids in the insulin molecule.

Intermediate-acting insulin begins working one to three hours after injection, reaches peak in six to twelve hours, and is gone in eighteen to twenty-six hours. The action of intermediate-acting insulin is slower than short-acting insulin because substances have been added to the insulin to slow its absorption from under the skin, two of which are protamine and zinc. These additives give the insulin a cloudy appearance in the bottle.

Long-acting insulin begins working four to eight hours after injection, reaches its peak in twelve to eighteen hours, and continues to work for twenty-four to twenty-eight hours. The addition of zinc prolongs the action of long-acting insulin. Long-acting insulin can be used in combination with short-acting insulin so that one has to take only three injections a day: one combination before breakfast, short-acting insulin alone before lunch, and another combination before supper.

Insulin can be taken in a number of combinations, called a mixed dose, all of which are prescribed by your physician. When they are first diagnosed, many diabetics experience a trial-and-error period with insulin dosages until the proper balance is achieved. Mixed doses provide an early peak to cover a meal you have just eaten, as well as a long duration of activity to keep you covered throughout the day or night. The usual combination is regular insulin mixed with intermediate-acting or long-acting insulin.

You can buy short-acting and intermediate-acting insulin premixed by the manufacturer in various combinations. People usually consider this more convenient, and it is a great help for people with poor eyesight or who have trouble with manual dexterity.

Insulin is sold by a number of pharmaceutical companies under different trade names. The label on the bottle describes the type of insulin, its source (animal or synthetic), and the strength. Lilly and Novo Nordisk are the two major U.S. manufacturers, and each company produces insulin of all types.

When you are first diagnosed with Type I diabetes and are started on insulin, your physician will prescribe a dosage regimen. At the beginning, establishing the best regimen for you will be mostly trial and error, but soon you will get into a groove, and you should stick to that regimen until there is a reason to change it. It is crucial that you use the same amount of insulin at the same times every day.

Common Insulin Preparations

Short-Acting (Onset 1/2-4 hours)

Product	**Manufacturer**	**Strength**
Humulin Regular	Lilly	U–100
Humulin BR (for pumps)	Lilly	U–100
Novolin R	Novo Nordisk	U–100
Novolin R Penfil	Novo Nordisk	U–100
Velosulin (human)	Novo Nordisk	U–100
Iletin II (beef)	Lilly	U–100
Iletin II (pork)	Lilly	U–100, U–500

Product	Manufacturer	Strength
Purified Pork R	Novo Nordisk	U–100
Velosulin (pork)	Novo Nordisk	U–100
Iletin I (beef, pork)	Lilly	U–40, U–100
Regular	Novo Nordisk	U–100
Iletin I Semilente	Lilly	U–40, U–100
Semilente	Novo Nordisk	U–100
Intermediate-Acting (Onset 1–4 hours)		
Humulin L	Lilly	U–100
Humulin N	Lilly	U–100
Insulatard Human NPH	Novo Nordisk	U–100
Novolin L	Novo Nordisk	U–100
Novolin N	Novo Nordisk	U–100
Novolin N Penfil	Novo Nordisk	U–100
Iletin II (beef)	Lilly	U–100
Iletin II NPH (beef)	Lilly	U–100
Iletin II (pork)	Lilly	U–100
Iletin II NPH (pork)	Lilly	U–100
Insulatard NPH	Novo Nordisk	U–100
Purified Pork Lente	Novo Nordisk	U–100
Purified Pork N	Novo Nordisk	U–100
Lente Novo	Nordisk	U–10
Iletin I Lente	Lilly	U–40, U–100
Iletin I NPH	Lilly	U–40, U–100
NPH	Novo Nordisk	U–100
Long-Acting (Onset 4–6 hours)		
Humulin U	Lilly	U–100
Iletin II PZI (beef)	Lilly	U–100
Iletin II PZI (pork)	Lilly	U–100
Iletin I PZI	Lilly	U–40, U–100

Product	Manufacturer	Strength
Iletin I Ultralente	Lilly	U–40, U–100
Ultralente	Novo Nordisk	U–100
Mixtures		
Mixtard	Novo Nordisk	U–100
(30% Short-Acting, 70% Intermediate-Acting)		
Mixtard Human 70/30	Novo Nordisk	U–100
(70% Intermediate-Acting, 30% Short-Acting)		
Novolin 70/30	Novo Nordisk	U–100
(70% Intermediate-Acting, 30% Short-Acting)		
Novolin 70/30 Penfill	Novo Nordisk	U–100
(70% Intermediate-Acting, 30% Short-Acting)		
Humulin 70/30	Lilly	U–100
(70% Intermediate-Acting, 30% Short-Acting)		

Insulin in Type I Diabetes

Type I diabetes develops in stages. When you are newly diagnosed, you may still have some, but not enough, beta cells in your pancreas that produce insulin. However, for the weeks or months prior to the diagnosis, you were insulin deprived, which is why you had symptoms. For this reason, you will probably need high doses of insulin to get your body working normally again. Your physician will make a decision about initial dose based on the number of beta cells still functioning, your body weight, and your level of physical activity. Once your blood glucose has come down to near normal levels, your dosage plan will even out.

The next stage of Type I diabetes is called remission, during which your diabetes appears to subside. It has not gone away; rather, your body is experiencing a reaction to finally having sufficient insulin after a long period of too little or none. During this period, you can probably get by with very small doses, but you should not stop taking insulin. If you do, you will need to start again, and you run the risk of developing an allergic reaction to insulin.

During the third stage, known as intensification, your few remaining beta cells are slowly destroyed by your immune system, and you no longer produce any insulin yourself. This results in a gradual rise in blood glucose, and your physician will increase your insulin dose in stages.

The final stage, called total diabetes, is reached when all the beta cells have been destroyed. This is when you settle down to your "final" dose regimen, usually three injections a day of a mixed dose of short-acting and intermediate-acting insulin. Although your schedule may differ slightly, the usual regimen is the following: a mixed dose taken about a half hour before breakfast, so that the insulin begins to work at about the same time you eat; another dose, this time of regular insulin, about thirty minutes before dinner; and an injection of intermediate-acting insulin before bedtime.

Insulin in Type II Diabetes

The vast majority of Type II diabetics get along fine on diet and exercise alone or with the addition of oral hypoglycemic agents. However, in certain instances, the diabetes may worsen. This may occur because the beta cells are reduced in number or are less effective or because of an increased tendency of other cells to resist using insulin. If this happens, you may need insulin injections, temporarily or permanently, depending on the cause. The amount of insulin needed varies widely from person to person and can change as time passes. Only your physician can determine how much insulin you will need and how often you will have to take injections.

For most Type II diabetics on insulin, standard therapy is twice-daily combinations of short-acting and intermediate-acting insulin. However, intermediate-acting insulin often wears off during the night, resulting in a before-breakfast blood glucose elevation that's difficult to control. This is especially true if it is taken before dinner. Since intermediate-acting insulin usually peaks fairly high, increasing the evening dose can result in hypoglycemia during the night. Therefore, many physicians now recommend a dose of long-acting (Ultralente) insulin at bedtime. This reduces the risk of nighttime hypoglycemia, and because Ultralente insulin has a longer action, it controls fasting blood glucose and can cover insulin needs at breakfast.

Probably the worst part about Type II diabetics needing insulin is the feeling of "failure," of not having been "good enough" to control the disease without insulin. You weren't "bad" or "wrong" in the way you were controlling your diabetes, but it doesn't feel that way. It feels like a step backward—or forward into worsening of the disease.

In a physiologic sense, this is true, but you have not mismanaged the disease. It's the fault of your pancreas. If you remain careful with your diet and exercise—and now your injections of insulin—and if you continue to keep your blood glucose at normal levels, you are no more in danger of contracting complications than you were before you went off oral hypoglycemics and onto insulin.

Taking Insulin

The thought of giving themselves an injection makes many people curl their toes and squeeze their eyes closed. "No way!" is the reaction when told that they are going to stick a needle into their own bodies every day—three times a day.

This is understandable. No one likes shots, and practically everyone turns their head when the nurse jabs a needle into their arm. It's a perfectly human reaction. But you will learn to do it, and in no time, you'll be preparing and giving yourself insulin injections with no more thought than you would give to taking a pill.

The first thing you need to know to make you feel less squeamish is that a shot of insulin is not the same as a shot of penicillin. There are three ways substances can be injected into your body: intravenously, meaning into a vein (such as emergency or slow-drip medications); intramuscularly, meaning into the muscle (such as a shot of penicillin); and subcutaneously, meaning under the skin (such as insulin).

In a subcutaneous injection, the needle is much shorter (about a half inch) and never reaches beyond the fatty tissue in the underlayers of skin. Some are even prelubricated, but they're more expensive and probably unnecessary since the needles are extremely fine and sharp. They do not puncture your muscles, veins, or arteries. (The little drop of blood that you'll see comes from the tiny capillaries near the surface of the skin.) Insulin syringes come in various sizes; you need to match the size to the dose so you can fit the entire dose into one syringe. Almost all insulin manufactured in the United States is U-100; you won't have a problem. Buy one hundred-unit syringes.

There are a number of elements in giving oneself insulin injections. A diabetes educator or other health professional in your physician's office will probably teach you how to do it, but here are the general guidelines:

- **Site selection.** Different parts of your body absorb insulin at different rates (in ascending order: abdomen, arms, thighs, and hips), so it's a good idea to develop a site rotation schedule. For instance, use the abdomen or arm in the morning when you need the quickest absorption and the thigh or upper buttocks in the evening when the insulin has to last all night. Rotating the site of injection also prevents a mound of tough, fibrous tissue (called hypertrophy) that would develop if you used the same site all the time. Eventually you'd have a hard time getting the needle in.
- **Preparing insulin.** Roll the bottle of cloudy insulin between your palms (no need to do this for clear insulin) and wipe off the rubber-stopper top with an alcohol swab. Draw air into the needle-tipped syringe by pulling the plunger out to the dose mark. Insert the needle through the rubber stopper and push in the plunger to force the air into the bottle. Turn the bottle upside down, making sure that the tip of the needle is in fluid (not air), pull the plunger again until the syringe is filled with insulin to your dose mark. Take the needle out of the bottle.
- **The injection.** Select the site, wipe the skin with an alcohol swab, and take a pinch of skin between your thumb and forefinger. Hold the syringe like a pencil in your other hand and push the needle straight into the skin. If you exhale and then insert the needle immediately after, your hand will be calmer and steadier. Push down on the plunger until all the insulin has been injected and remove the needle as you press down on the skin next to it with the alcohol swab.
- **Caring for and storing insulin.** Keep unopened bottles of insulin in the refrigerator (in the butter or egg compartment for handiness) but don't freeze it. You should always keep at least one extra bottle of each type of insulin on hand. Bottles you are currently using may be stored at room temperature, but keep them out of direct sunlight and away from radiators or heat registers. Do not store them near ice or let them freeze. Two

convenient places to store them are in your medicine cabinet or in your bedroom dresser. Always note the expiration date, and don't keep a bottle of opened insulin for more than a month, regardless of the expiration date. It will lose its effectiveness.

- **Maintaining supplies.** Disposable syringes are designed to be used once and thrown away. However, in order to save money, some people use a syringe two or three times. This is fine as long as you replace the cap on the needle after each use, use it again within twenty-four hours, and keep it in a safe place and away from children.
- **Needle safety.** Dispose of syringes and needles safely, for instance in a tightly covered can or jar that you keep in a closed cabinet out of the reach of children. When the container is full, tape it shut and put it out with your recycling or trash, whichever way your municipality requires. Never put loose needles in your trash or recycling bin.

An ordinary insulin syringe is not the only way to get the substance into your bloodstream, although it is the least expensive, and all Type I diabetics should learn to give themselves shots. A number of other devices are now on the market. An automatic injector works like the instrument used to obtain a drop of blood for glucose monitoring. It uses an ordinary syringe which is then loaded into a spring-cocked injector. After the site has been cleaned with alcohol, you place the injector next to the skin and touch the trigger, causing the needle to enter the skin; then you depress the plunger to push the insulin under your skin.

Other devices meet special needs. A jet injector does not use a needle at all, but rather forces insulin through the skin by means of air under pressure. For people with poor eyesight, there are various devices that audibly click when measures of insulin have been drawn up into the syringe and injected. Insulin pumps, which you may have heard about, will be discussed in chapter 9.

A pen injector looks like a fountain pen, with a disposable needle instead of a writing nib and a cartridge of insulin instead of a cartridge of ink. They are prefilled with 150 units of a variety of types of insulin, and you give yourself the amount you need, dispose of the needle, and put the pen injector back into your pocket or purse. They are excellent for multiple dose schedules and for people who are away from home and don't want to carry around a vial of insulin.

Other Medications Taken by Diabetics

Antihypertensives

Antihypertensive drugs lower blood pressure and are very commonly prescribed. They work in a number of ways: by dilating blood vessels so more blood reaches the heart; by blocking certain nerve receptors that control blood pressure; by depressing specific cardiovascular centers in the brain; by depressing or inhibiting the action of certain neurotransmitters (chemicals that send messages along nerve pathways); and by helping the body excrete sodium, which in turn increases elimination of excess body fluids.

There are dozens of antihypertensive drugs on the market today; some of the most commonly prescribed are Aldochlor, Aldomet, Apresoline, Cardizem, Esidrix, Esimil, Hydrodiuril, Inderal, Inderide, Lopressor, Minipress, Procardia, Serpasil, Tenex, Vasotec, and Wytensin.

For the most part, all these drugs can be taken safely with insulin and oral hypoglycemic agents. The only note of caution is for people who take diuretics, especially drugs that contain thiazide preparations, which tend to elevate blood glucose. If you are taking thiazide diuretics, be sure to keep a particularly close watch on your blood glucose.

Cholesterol-Lowering Drugs

Many people whose blood glucose levels have been elevated for a longer-than-normal period of time also have elevated cholesterol levels. If blood cholesterol cannot be controlled by diet alone, your physician may prescribe a cholesterol-lowering drug such as Mevacor, Zocor, Pravachol, or Lipitor. They can be taken safely with insulin and oral hypoglycemics.

Arthritis and Pain Medications

Osteoarthritis is extremely common among older people; in fact, the older you are, the more likely you are to have some degree of arthritis, which is the inflammation of joints. The two major symptoms are pain and reduced range of motion, both of which can be significantly relieved by a relatively new class of medication:

nonsteroidal anti-inflammatory drugs such as Naprosyn, Motrin, Feldene, Indocin, Nuprin, Toradol, and many others.

Many people with arthritis also take over-the-counter pain relievers such as aspirin, acetaminophen, buffered aspirin, aspirin or acetaminophen in combination with caffeine and/or phenacetin, and ibuprofen. All can be taken safely with insulin and oral hypoglycemics.

Cough and Cold Medications

Even though you can't cure a cold or the flu (you just have to wait patiently for it to go away on its own), everyone wants relief of the symptoms. The variety of products on the market for this is so big and changes so often that it would not be productive to list them here. With one exception, they can be taken safely with insulin and oral hypoglycemics. The exception is drugs containing ephedrine, which elevates blood glucose. Ephedrine is one of the most common ingredients in cold remedies that clear nasal passages (Neosynephrine, for example), so if you must unblock your stuffy nose, read the label carefully and take the lowest possible dose of ephedrine and monitor your blood glucose twice as often as you usually do. If it rises precipitously, stop taking the drugs and suffer through your stuffy nose, or steam yourself into greater comfort.

Minerals and Diabetes

Recently, there has been much discussion in the mainstream medical press about the role of four metallic elements in the treatment of diabetes. However, regardless of how enticing the following sounds, there is no proof yet that taking supplements of any of these minerals will be of benefit to diabetics.

Chromium

Chromium is found in many body tissues as part of a compound called glucose tolerance factor (GTF), which appears to play a role in the metabolism and regulation of glucose. How it does this remains unknown, but it may help insulin bind to receptors on cells. Some researchers believe that a chromium deficiency may thus be a contributing factor in Type II diabetes.

Based on laboratory experiments on rats as well as humans, there is some evidence that taking small doses of chromium can improve insulin action and glucose metabolism, as well as protect against arteriosclerosis, but only in people with a chromium deficiency. In both rat and human experimental subjects, extra chromium had no effect on the glucose tolerance of healthy individuals who had sufficient chromium (Dinsmoor 1994).

Studies on diabetics have been conflicting. Some people showed improved glucose tolerance when given two hundred micrograms a day of chromium, and some did not. Other studies have shown that chromium can elevate levels of high-density lipoprotein ("good cholesterol") in both diabetic and nondiabetic people—but only those who were chromium deficient to begin with (Dinsmoor 1994).

There is also some evidence that Americans in general are chromium deficient because the average diet is high in refined sugar, which tends to cause the loss of chromium through the urine. Chromium levels tend to decrease with age as well. However, the deficiency is not severe, and there is still no proof that it plays any role at all in diabetes.

Magnesium

Magnesium is a component of bone, other body tissues, and enzymes. Most people have sufficient magnesium—except diabetics, almost 40 percent of whom suffer from a deficiency of this mineral (Dinsmoor 1994).

There may be a relationship between magnesium deficiency and diabetes, but no one knows what it is—if it indeed exists. Diabetes appears to affect normal use of magnesium, which is excreted through the urine. People with high blood glucose tend to urinate more than normal, and they sometimes have impaired kidney and intestinal function, which also contribute to magnesium loss. Moreover, low-calorie diabetic diets may not provide sufficient magnesium. Low magnesium also may be a risk factor for cardiovascular disease and development of diabetic retinopathy.

Magnesium in turn may further aggravate poor blood glucose control by interfering with insulin secretion and increasing insulin resistance. Some studies show that giving magnesium supplements to both elderly nondiabetics and people with Type II diabetes significantly improved secretion and action of insulin. The recommended daily intake of magnesium is 400 mg, which is easily derived from green leafy vegetables, nuts, peas, beans, and whole grain cereal.

Zinc

Zinc levels are a factor in many body functions, including use of insulin. Some laboratory animals with diabetes have a zinc deficiency, but no one knows how many people, diabetics especially, have too little zinc. Increased urination and impaired intestinal absorption may promote zinc deficiency, but no one really knows. In laboratory experiments on rats, zinc deficiency has been associated with decreased insulin secretion and increased insulin resistance, but adding zinc to the rats' diets had no effect on glycohemoglobin levels.

You should be getting 15 mg a day of zinc, which is available from lean meat, seafood, milk, eggs, whole grain bread, and cereal.

Vanadium

Compounds of vanadium, a trace element that occurs naturally in plants and animals, seem to have insulin-like properties. Two of these compounds, vanadate and vanadyl, appear to normalize blood glucose levels in laboratory animals with Type I and Type II diabetes. Vanadate and vanadyl increase the transport of glucose into fat and muscle cells, increase glucose metabolism, speed up conversion of glucose into glycogen (the form in which glucose is stored), and slow the breakdown of fat. However, no one knows how they do this.

Various trials in humans are now underway to determine if giving people vanadium compounds can decrease their need for insulin.

6

Professional Help

Creating Your Own Diabetes Team

Many diabetes books use the phrase "diabetes team" as if there were a group of people, all wearing white coats with stethoscopes dangling from their necks, huddled around a conference table with serious expressions, discussing you and your disease. This is a nice fantasy (you might want to put in some cheerleaders if you're especially creative), but it's generally not true. There are a number of different physicians and health care providers you will see over the years, and some of them may speak on the telephone once in a while about a part of your care, but they do not generally have much contact with each other.

In fact, you will have to take the lion's share of coordinating various aspects of your care. Although physicians generally have your best interest at heart and they do care about how well you are managing your diabetes, it is your responsibility—as the person most invested in your health—to manage your own care. Your primary care physician and your endocrinologist may be the only ones who know you when you show up at the office; because you see specialists less frequently, they are less familiar with your case, making it all the more important that you advocate for yourself.

This is not to say that physicians are cold and callous, but the practice of medicine has changed drastically in the past decade and will change even more in the future, as managed care programs attempt to reduce escalating health care costs to increase their profits. You probably have noticed many of the changes, including more crowded waiting rooms, longer delays, more emphasis on insurance or prepayment, and more office assistants doing simple medical tasks (such as taking blood pressure).

For these and other reasons, you need to be ready to assert yourself and make certain that you receive the care you need. If you do not, you have the right and responsibility to change physicians; don't forget, you are the paying customer.

> *Betty allowed herself to be maltreated by incompetent doctors for almost three years. When she was first diagnosed, the physician she was seeing didn't know the difference between Type I and Type II, but that wasn't what bothered her. She changed doctors because she continued to feel awful for about eight months after she—and her physician—knew she had diabetes.*
>
> *During that time, Betty never went to a library or bought a book about diabetes, though she herself was an educator. She found a low-sugar cookbook and changed her eating habits, which helped a little, though it didn't occur to her while she was in the bookstore to go over to the health book section and find something on diabetes.*
>
> *Betty's second physician, an internist, confirmed her diabetes and told her to "watch her sugar." He never instructed her to buy a blood glucose monitor, never mentioned the importance of monitoring, never referred her to a diabetes educator or a nurse practitioner, and never gave her a food plan to follow.*
>
> *She tried to take care of herself by losing weight. However, she has Type I and is very slim, so she didn't actually need to lose weight. She lost a total of about thirty pounds over the next year and a half while she was with this internist, but she still didn't feel right. She still made no attempt to learn about diabetes.*
>
> *Finally, a friend got on her case and practically dragged her to an endocrinologist, and Betty's been with her ever since. She put Betty on insulin and helped her develop a food plan. She feels much better now, especially since she started using an insulin pump.*

Betty could have saved herself years of ill health by reading up on diabetes and taking her care into her own hands. Her situation shows the danger in placing all responsibility into the hands of physicians, who are at best very busy and at worst potentially incompetent.

Following are the health care practitioners who comprise your diabetes "team":

- A primary care physician is your regular doctor. They are usually family practitioners or internists and treat you for all ailments and general health care that does not require surgery or another specialist. This is the person you will see most often, and in a large group practice or one that has many elderly people, there may be a diabetes educator on staff. If you are a Type II diabetic, your diabetes is well-controlled on diet alone or diet and oral hypoglycemic agents, and you suffer no complications of diabetes, you probably won't need to see anyone other than your primary care physician.
- A diabetes specialist (endocrinologist), also sometimes called a diabetologist, is a physician who deals with diseases of endocrine glands. Most endocrinologists are knowledgeable about diabetes care, but some specialize in other endocrine glands, so when you call for an appointment ask about their experience with diabetes. You will need to see an endocrinologist if you have Type I diabetes, which is usually more difficult to manage; if you have trouble controlling you blood glucose; or if you develop a complication.
- A geriatrician is a physician who specializes in health problems of the elderly. You may not be ready for a geriatrician's services now, but since you will have diabetes for the rest of your life, you will be sooner or later. And if you have been diagnosed with diabetes for the first time after age sixty, you may want to seek the services of a geriatrician right away, especially if your physician is not experienced in caring for elderly diabetics.
- A registered dietician, also called a nutritionist, is a health care professional who assesses your nutritional needs, preferences, and lifestyle and then develops a food plan to meet those needs within the bounds of diabetic requirements. They generally know more about the relationship between food and diabetes than the other specialists listed here. If you can manage to plan meals and follow your own food plan to keep your blood glucose in control, you may not need to see a dietician,

but if you have any trouble at all you should make an appointment to see one. It is also a good idea to have at least one consultation with a dietician when you are first diagnosed—and again in a year or two to make certain you stay on track.

- A psychologist is someone to see when you need mental health counseling. A psychologist holds a Ph.D. and performs many functions (testing, administration, research), but you will want to find one who specializes in clinical treatment, that is, working directly with patients both individually and in groups. If you have negative feelings about seeing a mental health professional, try to remember that the strongest people realize and acknowledge when they need help.
- A clinical social worker is also a mental health counselor. They hold a Master of Social Work degree and have training in providing direct patient care. Social workers often do not have the depth of theoretical background that psychiatrists and psychologists do, but most of them have the advantage of seeing life as a series of problems to be solved and are therefore more likely to see your feelings as situational rather than as pathological.
- A pharmacist is the person who fills your prescriptions. If you patronize a large chain drugstore or supermarket pharmacy, you probably won't even see the pharmacist, but you can if you want to. Most are more than willing to answer your questions, either in person or on the phone, about your diabetes medication. It is a good idea to go to the same pharmacy to have all your prescriptions filled because many have your information in their computer system so they can be automatically warned of dangerous drug interactions. Nevertheless, you should still tell your physicians about all the drugs you are taking.
- An ophthalmologist is a physician who specializes in eyes and is one of the most important people you will see. You should have a dilated eye examination at least once a year, and you should tell your ophthalmologist as soon as your diabetes is diagnosed. Do not confuse an optometrist (who does cursory eye exams and makes eyeglasses) or an oculist (makes eyeglasses only) with an ophthalmologist. Go only to the latter for an eye exam.
- An exercise specialist is a person who can devise an exercise program appropriate to your lifestyle, food intake, and physi-

cal abilities. Most diabetics do not need the services of such a person, but your physician will recommend one if you choose.

- A certified diabetes educator (often a nurse practitioner) is someone trained in teaching patients and their families about diabetes, providing guidance for managing the disease and answering questions that crop up, especially in the beginning. If your physician does not have a diabetes educator on staff, you may ask for a referral. Most hospitals have diabetes educators.
- A podiatrist is a doctor (not a physician) who cares for feet. Diabetics need to take special care of their feet, which can be affected by peripheral neuropathy. If you develop foot problems, such as bunions, corns, and ingrown toenails, go to a podiatrist; do not attempt to treat yourself.

What a Professional Monitors

Although you bear most of the responsibility for keeping yourself healthy and managing your diabetes, there are certain things you need a health professional to do for you. These include routine blood tests (blood lipids [fats], cholesterol and triglycerides [HDL and LDL], thyroid function, and glycohemoglobin); urinalysis; dilated eye examination; retinal photographs, if necessary; blood glucose; and blood pressure (even if you monitor your own blood pressure, your physician should check it with more sensitive equipment).

Glycohemoglobin, also called glycosylated hemoglobin, hemoglobin A1c, or HbA1c, is a test that measures overall diabetes control. Here's how it works: As glucose circulates in the blood, it is attached to proteins. The more glucose in the blood, the more proteins carry it. Hemoglobin is a protein in red blood cells that carries oxygen from the lungs to all cells of the body. If the hemoglobin has glucose attached to it, it is called glycohemoglobin. The glycohemoglobin test shows average blood glucose over three months—the life of a red blood cell. The test provides accurate information about how well you are controlling your diabetes; it makes "allowances" for occasional high or low blood glucose because it measures average glucose over a fairly long period of time. Results of the test can give you excellent guidance on how well you have been doing and/or what changes you might make in diabetes management. You should have a glycohemoglobin test at least every six months (more if your physician recommends it).

Relationships with Health Care Providers

Although a health care provider is legally and morally bound to take care of your health, you are the only one who can—for the most part—determine if this is being done appropriately. Some things you have no control over, but you will be surprised at how much you can control.

Don't forget that choice is a powerful tool. You choose your physicians, and you choose to stay with them or find someone else. Most people find a physician through referrals from friends or relatives. If you are new to an area, ask around to find a doctor who people seem satisfied with. Ask yourself what's important to you in a physician: gender, age, office location, office hours, personality, type of practice (solo or group—although you won't find the former much anymore).

Trust and respect are integral parts of the patient-physician relationship. These develop (or don't develop) over time, but you can get a fairly good idea during your first visit of how the physician practices. Many people like to make the first visit a conversation only (sort of like interviewing the physician for the very important job of caring for your health), during which you state what you require from the physician and ask about practice guidelines. You can do this with a primary care physician and a specialist.

Find out how long you will generally have to wait in the office. My doctor is chronically late (and her office staff are chronically nasty). When I complained about both, she ignored the latter and told me that I will have to get used to her being late; it was the way it would always be in her office. So I had a decision to make; I had to weigh the fact that I liked the physician and considered her an excellent practitioner against the irritation of sitting in her office. I ameliorated the problem by always making the first appointment in the morning. She is still late, but my waiting time was cut way down. I try to ignore the office staff, and when something particularly egregious happens, I complain in writing.

Ask for what you need. Each time you visit your physician, make a list of things you want to discuss and questions you want answered and don't leave until you are satisfied. Be sure you stay informed about your diabetes and the rest of your health care. Ask for (and request an explanation of) the various tests your physician does, and make certain you understand what is said. If the physician treats your concerns lightly (or doesn't return phone calls), you may choose to leave the practice. But don't leave until you have a new physician and can get your records transferred.

Health care is a two-way street. You have responsibilities, too. You are the only one who knows how you feel and you are the one with the diabetes. You must make every effort to control your diabetes, keep accurate records when appropriate, take your medication as directed, take care of your body, make appointments for your required check-ups, and be honest about what is going on in your life.

Following are some reasons why you may decide to leave a medical practice:

- The physician doesn't listen or pay attention to what you are saying or doesn't make notes in your medical record about what you say and feel.
- Your questions aren't answered to your complete satisfaction, or when your physician answers questions or explains things, you don't understand the language.
- You never find out why you need a certain test or procedure or medication, and your doctor doesn't tell you the dangers and negative effects of procedures and medicines.
- You feel rushed through the visit, and the physician is too busy to give you all the time you need.
- The physician doesn't return phone calls.
- The physician seems intoxicated or distracted.
- The physician refuses to make accommodations about money by reducing the amount of the bill if you are short of funds, or allowing you to pay off the bill a little at a time.
- The physician becomes belligerent or defensive if you say you want a second a opinion, object to a certain treatment, or ask what the alternatives are to a recommended treatment. (Remember, it's your health at stake, and you always have the final word.)

If you decide to leave your physician, don't do it until you have found another one. A physician is obligated to treat you as long as you are a patient (refusal to do so is considered patient abandonment and is unethical and illegal), but once you leave the practice, that obligation ceases. So don't leave yourself in the lurch. You never know when an emergency will crop up.

The Diabetic Manifesto

A new national organization, Diabetics Educating and Empowering Diabetics (DEED), founded by Roy A. Flowers, has created a document that, if followed by all diabetics and the people who provide their health care, would prevent many of the problems in the doctor-patient relationship. It would also go a long way toward improving diabetic care. The full document, written and copyrighted by Flowers, is available from DEED (301-972-0617). Following are its points most pertinent to the doctor-patient relationship:

The Diabetic Manifesto

I have diabetes mellitus, a serious medical condition for which there is no cure. I must assume certain responsibilities or suffer the consequences. I must learn to control my diabetes and strive to normalize my blood glucose or face diabetes-related complications such as blindness, kidney failure, heart attack, stroke and neuropathy.

As a responsible person, I realize these consequences are not mine alone—I have a responsibility beyond myself to manage my condition. As a beneficiary of my increased responsibility, I expect society to help me obtain the tools and education I need to manage my condition.

As a person with diabetes, I have the following rights:

- *I have the right to expect the same consideration as other human beings. I expect others to respect my decisions about what is best for me. I expect others to accept me as a person and not as a treatment regimen. It's not acceptable for others to make judgmental statements because I'm on multiple injections or because I find I can no longer control my diabetes by diet and exercise alone.*
- *I have rights as a health care consumer. I reserve the right to make changes in my health care team when they fail to meet my needs. I expect access to diabetes specialists who will help me manage my health care team. I expect access to nutritional and exercise instruction necessary to aid in the management of my condition.*

- *I am the consumer and expect to be fully involved in my personal health care. I expect health care providers to include me in the decision-making process surrounding my diabetes management. I expect clear and concise explanations for all treatment regimens, including the reason for the treatment, the expected result, possible side effects, dose, frequency, and timing. I expect to be asked for my input into treatment plans created for me. I expect to be asked if I can conform to such a plan or if I have suggestions that will make conformance more realistic for me. I expect full access to my medical records, including copies of test results with concise verbal explanation of their meaning.*
- *I understand that the DCCT and similar studies have demonstrated the value of tight blood glucose control for prevention of complications and the extension of life. I expect health care providers to prescribe treatment regimens that aggressively pursue tight blood glucose control. I expect regular glycosylated hemoglobin measurements as part of diagnostic testing.*
- *I expect my physician and health care team to understand and keep abreast of new treatment modalities for diabetes. I expect regular visits to an endocrinologist at no greater than three-month intervals, and I expect to receive yearly assessments of my eyes, thyroid, kidneys, heart, and nerves.*
- *I expect health insurance and managed care organizations to underwrite the costs of treatments and supplies in support of tight blood glucose control.*
- *I have a responsibility to myself. I must assume management of my disease; I must become my own primary caregiver. I must learn as much as I can about diabetes and its treatment so that I can make informed decisions. I must seek the help and support of others before my ability to cope becomes critical.*

7

Self-Management

Diabetes Is for Life

Diabetes will be with you for the rest of your life, but if you take care of yourself, it won't necessarily shorten your life or make it less enjoyable. The disease is not curable, but it is definitely controllable. You are the one who will control it. And if I've said it once, I'll say it a thousand times: Maintaining normal blood glucose levels is the single most important way to control your diabetes. This is not simply a harangue from physicians and diabetes educators; it has been scientifically proven over the years.

Following are the blood glucose goals you ought to keep in mind:

Time of Measurement	Acceptable Range
Fasting	60–120 mg/dl
One hour after a meal	80–180 mg/dl
Two hours after a meal	70–150 mg/dl
Three hours after a meal	60–130 mg/dl

Penny, who has Type II diabetes, said: "Type II is harder to deal with than Type I because many of us don't take it as seriously as we should." She has a point. All the Type I diabetics that I have met so far are extremely serious about testing their blood glucose and try to maintain as tight control as possible. They all take their insulin injections when they should, they all carry their glucose monitors and injection paraphernalia with them wherever they go. In fact, most of them seem obsessed with their disease. Jill, a Type I diabetic I interviewed for this book, was a little insulted when I used that word to refer to the amount of time she devoted to thinking about the disease. "We're not obsessed," she explained. "An obsession is something neurotic. We *have* to think about it all the time and plan ahead for meals and insulin injections. If we don't, we get into trouble." She too has a point.

Change As a Way of Life

Some things in your life are going to change now that you have diabetes, but some can stay the same. Two important tasks relative to change are deciding which is which and accepting that change comes from within. No one can force you to lose weight, stop smoking, or quit drinking, nor can anyone else make you follow a diabetic food, exercise, and medication program. You have the choice not to do anything, but you will have to face the consequences.

One way to begin is to look back at your past experiences with change. Everyone has had them. For instance, how did your life change when you graduated from high school or college and had to earn your own living? What were the changes that took place when you got married? Had children? What happened when one or both of your parents died? How were things different when your kids grew up and moved out of the house? If you have other chronic diseases, how did they change your life? These changes are big, they are permanent, and they have enormous emotional content attached to them. Just like diabetes.

So, when you and your physician and/or diabetes educator sit down to plan various aspects of your life, you have to think about change. For instance, you'll need to ask yourself how the type of work you do is going to affect the necessity to monitor blood glucose and take insulin. If you have an office job and no one pays any attention to you when you close your door or go to the bathroom, nothing there will change. You simply take your monitor and insulin apparatus with you to work and work around your diabetes schedule. But if you work on an assembly line or are in an environment where breaks are strictly controlled and watched, you will have to explain the situation to your supervisor and make sure that you are not penalized for taking time to do what you have to do.

You'll need to think about other aspects of your lifestyle. For instance, do you travel a great deal for work or pleasure? If so, there's no reason why you can't be on the go as much as ever, but you will have to make blood glucose testing and medication taking part of your travel planning. You'll have to think about diabetes more when you travel than you do at home, and this will be a significant change.

Consider your age and current level of fitness; this will make a difference in how able you are to get sufficient exercise. What are your food preferences? Are you a "cookie monster" who will have a great deal of trouble giving up sweets, and do you refuse to eat any low-fat foods? If so, you will have to make more significant dietary changes than someone who is already eating what amounts to a "diabetic diet" and can easily refuse dessert.

You also will need to consider how your diabetes will affect those you love. Do you live with family or a friend or lover, and how are they reacting to your diabetes and all the changes it is making in your life? Your relationship with them will probably change. This is not necessarily a bad thing, but you need to be prepared for it.

Quit Smoking

Smoking significantly increases the risk of long-term complications of diabetes, especially cardiovascular and kidney disease and neuropathy. You need to quit smoking. There are no two ways about it. Chances are you want to quit. You've been meaning to quit. You've promised yourself you'll quit on such-and-such a date. Now you will.

Up until now, you may have given yourself a million reasons not to. It's perfectly natural to be afraid to stop smoking. Questions swirl through your mind as you contemplate the anguish of giving up cigarettes. What if I try and fail? What if I really don't want to quit? What if I can't stand up to the withdrawal symptoms? What if I freak out and embarrass myself? All these questions are legitimate. You might not succeed on your first try. You like to smoke so of course you want to keep on doing something that is so pleasurable and meets so many of your needs. But you can't.

There are a number of techniques for quitting smoking, and you might want to read a few books on the subject or sign up for smoking cessation classes. It is not within the scope of this book to go into detail about the quitting process, but you should sit down today and look in the phone book for information (you may want to call the American Heart Association, the American Lung Association, or the American Cancer Society) or go to your local bookstore for books on the subject. You need to quit now.

Taking Care of Your Body

Foot Care

Foot complications are common among diabetics, especially Type I. In addition to problems arising from peripheral neuropathy (see chapter 9), there are other causes:

- There is a greater tendency toward blocked blood vessels, which decreases blood circulation to the extremities. Blood circulation is an important factor in wound healing. Signs of poor circulation include leg cramps, slow healing of scratches, redness of feet when you are sitting, abnormally sparse hair growth, and leg pain at night which can be relieved by hanging them over the side of the bed.
- Many Type II diabetics are overweight, which increases the strain and pressure on the feet. If you are very overweight, you may not be able to bend over sufficiently to inspect and care for your feet.
- If you have trouble seeing where you are going because you have eye problems, you are prone to accidents that affect your feet: cuts, bruises, stubbed toes, blisters, and the like.
- The higher risk of infection in diabetics creates exacerbation of what for a nondiabetic would be a minor nuisance. A diabetic has the potential to lose a foot over an unnoticed or untreated blister.
- Loss of sensation means that you may not be aware of foot injuries. You could walk for blocks with a stone in your shoe and not notice it.

The feet are especially vulnerable to infection in poorly controlled diabetics, and any little sore, cut, blister, abrasion, or other break in the skin should be attended to thoroughly and immediately. Wash the cut and the surrounding area with soap and water and apply a mild antiseptic. Apply a sterile dressing and keep off that foot as much as possible. Don't use old-fashioned cloth adhesive tape because when you pull it off, you also pull off a layer of skin. Use surgical tape instead; it is available in drugstores and supermarkets. Take off the dressing when you shower and reapply it with more antiseptic.

If the sore doesn't begin to heal or if it becomes infected, (draining pus or signs of hot, reddened skin around the sore) it requires medical attention. If your own physician cannot see you right away, go to an emergency room.

Following are all the things diabetics need to do for proper foot care:

- Wash your feet in warm (not hot), soapy water every day, but don't soak them. Soaking softens the skin too much and increases vulnerability to infection.
- After washing, lubricate your feet with an emollient cream (not oil), but don't rub any between your toes. If your feet perspire heavily, use an absorbent powder, but again, not between your toes where it can cake.
- Examine your feet every day. Use a good light and mirror to visualize the bottoms. You're looking for areas of dryness or scaliness, broken skin, ingrown toenails, and redness.
- Cut your toenails straight across and don't dig into the corners. If rough edges remain, use a nail file or emery board.
- Immediately care for corns, calluses, warts, and blisters. Don't tear off loose skin or pop blisters, and watch for redness and discoloration. In other words, don't do your own foot surgery; let a podiatrist take care of your feet and mention that you are diabetic.
- Don't let athlete's foot or other fungal infection go untreated. Use an antifungal cream and wear cotton or wool socks or one of the new synthetic materials that wick moisture away from your skin.
- Make certain your shoes are comfortable and fit well. Don't wear shoes that squeeze your toes or cramp your feet in any way. Very high heels may make women's legs look sexy, but they are terrible for the feet and you should switch to lower heels. Both diabetic men and women need to get rid of their pointy-toed shoes.

- Never go barefoot, even at home. Even on the beach, you should wear sandals of some sort. There are too many sharp stones and other objects around.
- Socks and stockings should have no seams, darns, or other things that can chafe and cause blisters. Wear clean socks (preferably wool or cotton) or stockings, and if they get wet from perspiration, rain, or stepping in a puddle, change them right away.
- Don't let your feet get too hot or too cold. Avoid frostbite at all costs.

Skin Care

Diabetics have the same skin problems as everyone else—and then some, especially if their diabetes is in poor control. First, their skin can become excessively dry. This can be counteracted by using skin lotions and emollients, but it is best to prevent it by good blood glucose control and drinking lots of water.

If you have high blood cholesterol, you might see orange-yellow fatty plaques (xanthomas) around your eyes or on shins and elbows. If you significantly lower your blood cholesterol, by diet alone or with the help of medication, they will disappear.

Necrobiosis lipodica diabeticorum (NLD) is a relatively harmless but unattractive condition in which the layer of fat beneath the skin is destroyed. It makes the skin look thin, discolored, and dimpled. It occurs more frequently in female diabetics than in males and begins usually in adolescence. The most common site is the front of the shins. In itself, NLD is nothing to worry about, but you should be careful to protect the affected skin because it can easily break or tear and is especially vulnerable to injury. There is no treatment, and it often disappears in time.

The most important things diabetics can do for their skin is to take care of it, protect it from the elements, and treat it immediately and appropriately when it breaks. Take these precautions:

- Avoid sunburn. Always (not just when you go to the beach) use a sunblock on all exposed skin in summer, and do the same in winter if you are outdoors a lot. It may be cold out, but the glare of the sun can do a lot of damage as it bounces off ice and snow onto your skin.

- Wash your entire body every day with warm soap and water. If you prefer baths to showers, it is a good idea, before you leave the tub, to stand under the shower for a minute or two to rinse off the dirty bath water.

Weight Control

Beyond the fact that maintaining normal weight is one of the best ways to keep diabetes in control and prevent long-term complications, there is little further to say about weight control that we haven't already covered—and that you probably don't already know. You don't need another harangue about losing weight, but this might be a good time to turn back to chapter 3 to review techniques for losing weight.

Eye Care

You must take excellent care of your eyes, and the most important part of self-maintenance is to make an appointment for an annual dilated eye examination. Wash your hands whenever you touch your eyes, especially when you have a cold or the flu or when you have been in contact with someone who is ill. You should pay particular attention to cleanliness if you wear contact lenses.

If you spend a great deal of time reading or using a computer, take a short "eye break" every fifteen or twenty minutes: look away from your work and stare into the distance or close your eyes for a few minutes.

Urine Testing for Ketones

If your insulin level falls too low, your body will burn fat instead of carbohydrates. One product of fat burning is ketones, which are toxic. Therefore, it is important to detect their presence before the level has a chance to build up.

Since ketones are excreted in the urine, this is where you will test for them. The procedure is simple: You buy ketone test strips in a drugstore (some large supermarkets have them) and read the directions because different brands take different amounts of time to "develop."

You should test for ketones whenever the following occur: blood glucose reading of 240 mg/dl or more; when you are ill, especially if you are vomiting or have diarrhea; every day before breakfast during pregnancy; during acute psychological or physical stress; or when you have a fruity odor on your breath, have trouble breathing, or feel faint or dizzy.

If your ketone level is elevated, you must get it down to normal immediately. Give yourself an injection of the amount of regular insulin that your physician has prescribed for such an eventuality. If you have had no such instructions, call and find out. If it's after hours, tell the answering service that this is an emergency—because it is. Also, you should drink plenty of water to prevent dehydration and help flush the ketones out of your system. Don't exercise because you will burn more fat and thus increase ketone production.

Dental Care

Good dental care can prevent gum infection, abscesses, and other dental problems that result in elevated blood glucose. There are four main elements: proper brushing and flossing, filling cavities, treating and preventing abscesses and infections, and treating and preventing gum disease.

As soon as you are diagnosed with diabetes, visit your dentist (even if it isn't time for a regular check-up) and mention that you have diabetes. You should receive a complete oral examination and a thorough professional cleaning. Don't shirk this part of your responsibility. No one likes to go to the dentist (you don't like paying taxes either, but you do it), but dental care has changed so much in recent years that it's no longer as awful as it used to be. The drills are high speed and flushed with cold water so you don't have that "sawdust smell" and uncomfortable sensation of heat. For anything that's going to be painful, you get a nice shot of novocaine, and the needles are so fine that you hardly feel it going in.

I told my dentist that I'm a big baby about pain, so he makes certain to slide the needle in slowly. I've had some anxious moments at the dentist's office (mostly about what it's going to cost), but I've never been in pain. If your dentist hurts you, find another one.

Following are the things you need to do to take good care of your teeth:

- Brush at least twice a day, preferably after every meal.
- Floss once a day, making sure you get down to the gum line.
- Massage your gums once a day with a water-jet device or a rubber tip at the end of your toothbrush. This increases circulation to your gums and reduces the chance of gum disease and infection.
- Use tartar control, plaque-fighting toothpaste.
- If your gums bleed when you brush, you probably have gingivitis (inflammation of the gums), which is a minor problem but one that should be treated by your dentist before it turns into a major one.
- If you have a toothache, go to the dentist immediately; delay will always exacerbate the problem.
- See your dentist at least twice a year for professional cleaning and an oral examination.

Education

One of the most important ways in which you can take care of yourself is to learn as much as you can about diabetes. You don't have to enroll in medical school, but you do need to learn basic facts about controlling diabetes. You are reading this book now, an excellent step toward self-education. There are other books that are much more technical for those who have a scientific bent or simply want greater detail.

You should learn the diabetes vocabulary so you can understand what health professionals are saying. Many of them don't know how to talk in anything but "medicalese," and it's a nuisance to have to keep asking them to translate.

> *Victor is thirty-seven-years old and was diagnosed with Type II four years ago. He had all the classic symptoms and his father had Type II, so when he went to the doctor, he was pretty sure what the doctor would say.*
>
> *Ten years prior to his diagnosis, during a routine physical examination, Victor found out that his blood glucose was 130. His doctor just shrugged and said, "Your sugar's a little high," and that was that. He wishes now that he had gotten*

the diagnosis back then, because he would have started taking better care of himself.

But he has made up for lost time. He has high blood pressure and high cholesterol so he's become a virtual vegetarian. He also takes a lot of pills, but he feels great and his blood glucose is okay. His wife and children are behind him 100 percent. His food plan has not been a hardship, as they recognize that this is the way they should have been eating all along.

Victor joined the American Diabetes Association as soon as he was diagnosed, and because he is a "take-charge guy," he was soon running the support group in a major Washington, D.C. suburban community. He doesn't say much in the group meetings, but he does all the behind-the-scenes work and keeps the group going. "Diabetes is one of the ways I feel as though I can serve my fellow man," said Victor—and he practices what he espouses.

Penny described her initial reaction to the diagnosis: "This is going to sound strange, but I had a little feeling of excitement, like it was going to be a challenge to see if I could keep my glucose in control and eat the way I should."

The first thing Penny did was read everything she could about diabetes. She joined a support group and went to a series of classes at a local hospital, and she still goes to workshops twice a year. "I learned much more about diabetes from reading and going to my groups than I ever did from my doctor," she said. Penny is not the only one to have had this experience.

Support Groups

At some time during your life as a diabetic, you may want to participate in a support group or become active in a diabetes organization; therefore, knowing something about your disease will be helpful and make you feel like less of an outsider. You'll have to put forth a little effort to do this, but it's not impossible. As you learn to control your diabetes, and as you read various pamphlets or brochures, the terms will become part of your everyday vocabulary before you know it.

It is worth thinking about joining a diabetes education program or support group. The American Diabetes Association and diabetes clearinghouses can give you the names and phone numbers of such programs in your area. Also, almost all hospitals have various support and educational groups. Call one or several community hospitals or medical centers and ask for the diabetes educator. There are a number of advantages to participation:

- Getting together on a regular basis with other diabetics is both comforting and informative. You may not want to do this forever, but when you are first diagnosed, it can be very helpful.
- Reading books and other materials on your own is fine, but if you have questions, and you surely will, learning in a group gets them answered right away. You also derive benefit from questions that other people ask.
- There are tips and items of practical advice that you would never otherwise think to ask or tell about, but that come up when sharing your experiences.
- You can take advantage of other people's mistakes, which they usually discuss freely in groups.
- You can compare brands of insulin, syringes, glucose monitors, and other paraphernalia of diabetes.
- Other people have had experiences with health insurance companies that they will be willing to share with you—and you can tell your horror stories to people who are really interested.
- Diabetes experts usually run the programs and groups. They are there for you to pick their brains.

Be careful, though, about the type of support group you join, and know that if you don't like it or you don't feel comfortable, you don't have to stay. There are all kinds of groups. Some are composed of people who just like to sit around and complain. Some are so serious and information oriented that you feel like you're back in high school. Others provide no real diabetes information but are socially a lot of fun. Some groups are led by certified diabetes educators, and some leaders are diabetes experts but not formally trained and certified. Others are run under the auspices of a hospital or clinic, and some are just a group of diabetics who happened to find one another. Some emphasize the psychological problems of diabetes and some the physical.

8

Stress and Its Effect on Diabetes

Effects of Stress and Other Emotions

There is almost no strong emotion that does not have an effect on blood glucose—and vice versa. Stress, fear, excitement, anger, and all the other feelings that swirl through your mind and heart can increase or decrease the amount of glucose circulating in the bloodstream, regardless of what you have eaten, or how much and what type of medication you have taken. By the same token, excessively high or low blood glucose can cause various emotions all by themselves (irritability, elation, depression), regardless of whatever else is going on in your life.

Of course, these effects vary from person to person and even from time to time within the same person. But emotions are like that: Some days your boss's irritating habit of dropping into your office unannounced and peering over your shoulder while you work doesn't bother you much. Other days, you want to strangle your boss for it.

Then too, not all your emotional reactions and feelings will affect your blood glucose, and not all your fluctuations in blood glucose are caused by emotions. One of the most important things to learn in dealing with and controlling diabetes is to determine how you as an individual are affected. This takes a while, but with judicious and well-timed blood glucose monitoring, you will get the hang of it.

Stress increases the release of glucose from the liver into the bloodstream, but the effect of stress on blood glucose varies from person to person. It almost seems as if some people can waltz through life in a constant state of angst and their glucose remains steady as a rock, whereas others will go into wild glucose fluctuation at the slightest hint of a stressful situation. This is probably due more to personality type than to physical reaction, although the latter cannot be discounted. For instance, a person who looks ready to take off and buzz around the ceiling from stress may not *feel* the stress levels that we perceive in that person. And if you don't feel it, there is no "reason" for your liver and insulin receptors to react.

When diabetics are stressed, however, most have some degree of glucose reaction—for two major reasons. The first is biochemical: various hormones actually do kick in and react to the stress. The second is emotional. When you are stressed, some of your daily routine is upset and you tend to engage in behaviors that are not helpful to diabetes control: overeating or forgetting to eat, forgetting to test blood glucose, and neglecting doses of medication.

Diabetes as a Stressor

Having diabetes, in and of itself, is a stressor.

Joyce found that, for her, one of the worst things about having the disease is that it's inconvenient. She has to test her blood glucose seven times a day, and she doesn't always want to, especially if she's not in a place where it's convenient to do it.

She uses an insulin pump and likes it because it has given her much greater flexibility about when she can eat, though she finds the forty-six inches of plastic tubing to be a nuisance; it's forever falling into the toilet when she sits down.

Homer is extremely stressed out by his diabetes, but he creates more stress for himself than most people with Type I diabetes experience. He tests his blood glucose eight to ten times a day, twice what his physician suggested. He also keeps a record of what the test results are, what every morsel of food he puts in his mouth is (including a breakdown of all the nutrients the food contains), how he is feeling each time he tests, and what physical activity he has done between that test and the one before. There is no medical reason why Homer has to test his blood glucose so often; he does it because he worries constantly about his diabetes control—and the worry stresses him out even more. His diabetes is, unnecessarily, a huge stressor in his life.

When you begin to feel stressed about your diabetes, think about how much of what you are feeling is necessary and how much is not. It is natural to experience stressful times, but diabetes is going to be with you for the rest of your life, so minimizing related stress and adopting a healthy, but not overwhelming, regimen is in your best interest.

Diabetes carries other stress factors: worry about how the blood glucose test is going to come out; anxiety about whether you'll be able to eat on time; dealing with awkward situations in social settings; having people treat you like a disabled person. All these things can be dealt with, of course, but doing so takes energy and creates stress.

Diabetes is always there. It is a chronic condition, and there is no way that it is ever going to go away. Some people adjust to this fact relatively quickly and some never do. The sooner you can, the better off you will be and the less stressful the fact of having diabetes will be. You don't have to like it—no one likes having a disease—but you do have to get used to it, and you do have to be realistic about doing what you must to take care of yourself. If you get annoyed and resent it every time you have to duck into the bathroom or close the door to your office to do a quick blood glucose test or give yourself a shot of insulin, you are going to be a very unhappy camper. A very stressed-out camper.

Because diabetes is entirely internal, you look like everyone else but you are not. There are, of course, other chronic diseases that don't have obvious physical manifestations, but diabetes is the most common and one of the most serious. So although you don't appear to be a person with a disease, you are, and you must be constantly engaged in controlling that disease. Some people find this stressful. It can be, and you certainly don't want to trivialize your diabetes, but again, you have to get used to it. One of the ways I have managed to do this, at least most of the time, is to realize that everyone has hidden problems that compromise their life and must be accommodated, and that a lot of those things are far worse than Type II diabetes in pretty good control.

Blood glucose can fluctuate for many reasons that are outside your control, and this can be frustrating and anger producing. Frustration and anger are powerful stressors. For example, you've been "good" for weeks, following your food plan, exercising, and monitoring your blood glucose on a regular schedule—and all of a sudden, you hit a snag and your blood glucose shoots up for no apparent reason. You do what you should to get it back in control, and in a few hours everything is all right, but the stress may linger, putting you at further risk of another episode of elevated blood glucose.

No matter how well you manage your diabetes, it is natural to worry about the future, about whether you will fall victim to a serious long-term complication. There's only one thing to do about this, and it sounds easier said than done, but you have to relieve yourself of this intense stress: Snap out of it!

Turn on the light, get out of bed, and turn on the TV or read a book. Roll over, wake your bed partner, and make love. If it happens during the day, do something other than what you were doing when the worry began to intrude on your thoughts. Go to a movie. Go to an art exhibit that you've been meaning to attend. Go shopping and buy yourself a special treat. Tell your boss you're not feeling well and leave work, and get out of the house if you are there all alone.

Stress Management in Daily Life

Assess the Stressors in Your Life

Some people hardly know they're under stress. They bite their fingernails, crack their knuckles, chew gum as if they were in the Olympic trials, and can't sleep more than two hours at a time. But when asked how they feel, they'll chirp, "Fine!" and never realize how stressed out they are. Then there are people who have to lie down for an hour (or tell three friends about it) if the cashier was rude to them in the supermarket or if a business colleague calls to change a lunch appointment at the last minute.

Most people can generally take things in stride, but on an off day, the least little thing can cause a major freak-out. Be prepared for these times and learn to recognize when you're feeling on edge. People have varying stress tolerance levels—from situation to situation and from time to time. This is perfectly normal. Your job is to learn to recognize the things that always get to you, as well as how you feel when even ordinary bumps in the day are hard to cope with.

Change is one of the things that most people find extremely stressful. Even a little thing like a new hairdo can affect your self-perception for a few days while you wonder if it looks good. But major changes create major stress, which can make blood glucose act like it's doing the jitterbug. Following are some of the things that create the most stress for most people, but remember that everyone is different so don't feel as though you "have" to get stressed out when one or more of these things happen. By the same token, you don't have to "grin and bear it" all by yourself. If you're having trouble coping, get some professional help. It's the mature, sensible thing to do.

- *A major personal loss.* The feeling of loss does not necessarily have to arise from death or divorce; when a close friend moves away, the pain can be as acute.
- *Being hurt in an automobile accident or other traumatic injury.* The more painful and long-lasting the injury, the greater the stress.
- *Life-threatening illness such as cancer or heart attack.* It is stressful when this happens to a loved one or to yourself.
- *Changing jobs.* This is stressful regardless of whether the change was your choice or that of your former employer. Being fired is not always more stressful than quitting.
- *Serious financial woes.* The stress is compounded when your house mortgage is foreclosed or your car is repossessed.
- *Pregnancy and birth or adoption.* This is a life-altering change that creates stress.
- *Trouble with the law.* Committing a felony and going to jail is more stressful than committing a misdemeanor and being fined, but both are awful.
- *A big promotion at work, or any significant personal achievement.* Again, stress does not have to be negative to be problematic.
- *Moving to a new house.* The act of moving in itself is stressful. However, if you move away from loved ones, especially if you're going to a town or city where you know no one, the level of stress may be even higher.

One other thing about assessing stress: Sometimes you can feel it even when you're not consciously aware of being stressed. If you're getting more headaches than usual, if you have a stiff neck or sore muscles for no reason, if you find that you're breathing rapidly and shallowly or grinding or clenching your teeth, or if you're suddenly tired all the time, you're probably under stress, and this would be a good time to look at what's going on in your life—and take steps to change what you don't like.

Develop a Positive Attitude

Developing a positive attitude is one of the most important things you can do, and it may be difficult to accomplish if you live and work in a highly stressful environment. So much of life is stressful that you have to concentrate on making your own private sphere as unstressful as possible. There are a number of ways to do this.

- Think about what you have control over and what you do not, and try to pay little or no attention to what you cannot control. For instance, if the shenanigans of the politicians in your city or state make you gnash your teeth, and you have no interest in becoming active in politics, don't read about them in the newspaper. If the murder rate is going up in your area, take reasonable precautions when you go out, but don't watch the blood and gore on the local news.
- Remember that you will not have total control over your diabetes all the time. It is by nature an unpredictable disease, and the best you can do is do your best. Once you learn and internalize this, you can stop feeling guilty and stressed out every time your blood glucose does something it's not "supposed" to.
- If you socialize with people you don't like or who are not congenial to be with, drop them. You needn't do it with insults; you don't even need to announce your intentions. Simply be unavailable when they call. There are enough unpleasant people in your life that you cannot drop (co-workers, grocery store clerks, family members); why should you voluntarily subject yourself to the stress of choosing to be with people you dislike?
- If your marriage or partnership is not as happy as you would like it to be, do something about it. Don't believe that you have

to suffer through another twenty or thirty years of misery. Talk honestly about your feelings to your partner, get into couple's counseling, or get out of the relationship.

- Try to increase your intuition and self-awareness and learn to identify what makes you happy and what does not. This requires conscious thought and a good deal of mental and emotional effort. I often practice it when I go for my walk. It's forty-five minutes of uninterrupted peace and quiet when I can devote myself entirely to myself.
- Learn to manage your own life. This is not to say that you should not develop close relationships with other people, and it is not to say that you should not allow other people to help you when you need it. But you, and only you, are responsible for the conduct of your own life—and the management and control of your diabetes.
- Recognize that there are choices to be made in every aspect of life. Too many people stay in jobs they hate or remain in unsatisfactory human relationships because they believe they have no choice in the matter. This is not true. Making choices and changes is often difficult and stressful, but in the long run, it is almost always less stressful than remaining in bad situations.
- Set short- and long-term goals in life that are realistic and achievable. Forcing yourself to do things that are impossible, pointless, or unnecessary is extremely stressful. You will probably never achieve the goal and will drive yourself crazy trying.
- Develop your sense of humor and laugh as much as you can. So much of life is absurd; try to see it.
- Become a volunteer and help others. Work for the homeless, volunteer at an animal shelter, read to nursing-home patients, participate in your local Meals on Wheels program, or tutor a child. It doesn't matter what it is, but do something for others.

Learn Relaxation Techniques

Meditation can take many forms. In its purest form, it is a Buddhist religious practice, but anyone can use the technique of meditation, and it need not be religious. It is a form of mental concentration that frees you from your usual mental processes. Some people say that meditation, if practiced consistently, can change your life.

Most people don't want to take meditative techniques that far; they just want a short mental vacation during the middle or at the end of a busy stressed-out day. Meditation does that by helping you to block out the outside world and taking you deep into your inner self.

The two types of Eastern meditation that are best known in the West are transcendental meditation (TM) and Zen meditation. The former constricts your attention when you repeat a word or a sound (mantra) over and over as you sit with your eyes closed. In Zen meditation, you sit with your eyes open and concentrate on your breathing.

General rules of meditation include doing it in the same quiet place every day when you will not be interrupted, preferably at the same time each day, and sitting in the full lotus or half lotus position. Meditating after eating or before going to bed is not recommended. Practitioners of meditation say you should start with brief periods—five minutes or so and gradually increase to twenty or thirty minutes. You should not skip days, and if you really think you don't have time to meditate, it is better to do it for only five minutes than not at all.

If you are going to practice TM, first choose your mantra, a short (no more than one or two syllables) sound that you hear as harmonious and melodious. Then go to your chosen spot, assume your position (if lotus or half lotus is too uncomfortable, just sit), take a few deep breaths to quiet yourself, close your eyes, and begin repeating your mantra over and over slowly and silently. If other thoughts come into your mind, don't push them away deliberately. Rather, let them flow through without letting up on your mantra concentration. Soon you will find yourself in a state of "suspended isolation" in which you neither think nor do. This is meditation. When you are finished, stop repeating your mantra, sit with your eyes closed for a few minutes longer and then open your eyes, stretch as you would when awakening, and go about your day.

Zen meditation requires that you use the full or half lotus position on the forward part of a straight chair. Your spine should be straight and the small of your back concave. Pull your chin in; and put your hands in your lap, thumbs touching, turned up with the left hand inside the right (opposite if you are left handed). With your eyes open but unfocused, look at a spot about three feet in front of you and downward. Move your torso in a wide arc back and forth a few times and stop at your natural center where you feel comfortable. Sit quietly and concentrate your mind on the rhythm of your breathing. As in TM, don't pay attention to the other thoughts that come into your mind; rather, concentrate on your breathing. You can count one-two as you inhale and exhale if it helps you concentrate, but soon you won't need to do even that.

Biofeedback

Biofeedback can reduce stress, or the symptoms of stress, by "proving" to yourself that certain mental exercises can lower your blood pressure, change your body temperature, calm your pulse, and ease muscle tension. In biofeedback, you are hooked up to electronic monitors that record these physical indicators of stress. As you do a variety of stress-reducing exercises, you can watch the monitor register the positive effects. The more you practice, the less you will need the monitor's proof of their effectiveness, and soon you will be able to do biofeedback at home without having to go to an instructor's office to be hooked up to the monitor.

There are a variety of ways you can learn biofeedback. Ask your physician to recommend an instructor, call the office of a physician who practices alternative healing techniques, call the American Association of Diabetes Educators at 800-338-3363, or ask a neurologist.

Pet Therapy

Pets are the most relaxing "people" you will ever have in your life. Dogs and cats provide unconditional love, they are always delighted to see you, and they don't care what you look like, whether your hair is combed, or if your makeup is fresh. They love lots of petting, stroking, and hugging, which is a known stress reducer (studies have shown that people who talk to and stroke their pets can lower their blood pressure).

People are often more likely to tell things to their pets than to the most intimate people in their lives, and pets, especially dogs, are always willing to listen. Cats sometimes need to be in another room, but they'll come around later to listen to what you have to say.

No matter how rotten a day you've had at work, the sight of a wagging tail and lolling tongue at the front door is bound to cheer you up. And the obligation to take your dog for a walk is also good for you. It's great exercise, and watching your dog sniff along, checking out who has been around his favorite bushes, is fun. They are so serious and intent as they go about their silly business that you can't help but smile. And the furry presence beside you or the tail wagging at the end of the leash ahead of you is extremely calming.

Cats probably invented the whole concept of relaxation; no creature on earth has perfected indolence as well as a well-cared-for cat. Just watching them lie stretched out in a patch of sunshine or curled up in a ball on your comforter makes you feel as though you'd like to do the same. Their soft luxurious fur calls out for gentle strokes, and when they are in the mood for a game, they're impossible to refuse, and there is no way you can think about anything else but the cat's antics.

If you are allergic to dog and cat dander, there are plenty of other choices. Gerbils, hamsters, and guinea pigs are a tremendous amount of fun and can be very affectionate. Rabbits are darling pets, very soft and huggable, and they can be litter box trained just like a cat.

Staring at a tankful of brightly colored tropical fish (and listening to the musical bubbling sounds of the water aerator) is incredibly relaxing. An increasing number of therapists have aquariums in their waiting rooms.

For people who live alone, a pet is practically essential. For old people or those who are recently widowed or divorced, a pet can mean the difference between misery and the ability to tolerate loneliness. Their presence in your life and the need to take responsibility for them can make all the difference.

Several years ago, my sweet orange tabby, Amanda, was in the hospital for five days. I thought she would die, but when the vet called to say I could come and pick her up, I burst into tears of joy. When I showed up at the animal hospital, the receptionist called out on the intercom: "Amanda Fromer, going home," and I cried again. It was the use of my last name as hers, corroborating what I have known all along: that she is family. When I heard her loud and happy meow as the nurse carried her (purring like crazy in anticipation) to the waiting room, it made my day.

Travel As a Source of Stress

Even if you are going on a much-needed and much-anticipated vacation, and even if you love to travel, it has its stressful moments. Will you make it to the airport on time? Will you make your flight connection? Will the weather be good for the car trip, will the kids be reasonably well-behaved this time, and will the transmission start acting up again? No matter how fabulous the scenery, how delightful the people, how awe-inspiring the art, you still have to think about your diabetes: monitoring your glucose, taking insulin or oral hypoglycemics, and making certain you get enough of the right kind of food.

Business travel is an almost guaranteed stressful event. You may not like the people you're traveling with, and even if you do, being with them constantly for a few days can put a strain on the best working relationship. You have goals to accomplish that are different from, and probably more stressful than, what you usually do at the office. You may be crossing a few time zones, which can wreak havoc on your eating and medication schedule. The hotel may be awful, and you may not be able to get your clothes pressed.

Also, much business travel involves food, and since sometimes the best deals are made in the best restaurants, you may have less control than you would like over where and what you eat. Moreover, alcohol tends to flow freely at business meals. The best advice here is follow your own rules for eating out (see chapter 3).

Does all this sound horrid? Some people think so and will do almost anything to avoid leaving home, but others take it in stride and enjoy even business trips. Frequent travelers have learned many of the things that make trips for diabetics easier to deal with. Here are some:

- Make certain you are healthy when you leave. You can't do anything about the cold you catch on the airplane from the viruses in the recirculated air, but if you are ill at home, stay at home until you feel better. Being sick on vacation can ruin your fun and make your diabetes really difficult to control.
- If you require immunizations for travel, get them at least a month before you leave so you have time to recover from reactions.
- Pack all the diabetic supplies and medication you will need for your trip—and then some—in your carry-on bag, never in checked luggage. Many frequent travelers recommend taking along twice as much as you expect to need. Ask your physician

for an extra prescription for all your medications and syringes in case you lose everything. Make sure the prescriptions have the generic name of the drug if you are planning foreign travel.

- Carry a supply of snacks. The best-laid travel plans have a habit of going awry, airplanes and trains are notoriously late, and meals can be delayed for hours. Not all airports have restaurants (or at least one you would want to eat in), and train stations usually limit you to a fast-food joint—if they have that.
- Call your health insurance company and make sure you are covered if you are traveling to a foreign country.
- Ask your diabetes educator or nurse practitioner what to do if you plan to cross two or more time zones. You will need to know how to adjust meals and medication for the change.
- The American Diabetes Association or the International Diabetes Federation can provide you with names of endocrinologists in areas where you will travel. If you do not do this beforehand and you fall ill while traveling, look in the yellow pages of the local phone book under either "diabetes" or "endocrinology" in the physicians section. Many hotels have doctors on call who can steer you to the right specialist, or in a real emergency, simply dial 911. If you are in a foreign country and have an American Express card, call the local office for a physician referral. Many Visa and MasterCard gold card memberships provide the same service.
- Take at least one travel companion into your confidence about your diabetes in case of an emergency.
- Wear a bracelet or necklace, or carry a notice in your wallet, that identifies you as a diabetic. It can be discreet, but it should be there. Also, in your wallet or some other conspicuous place, carry a notice of your allergies to medications, as well as the person(s) to notify in case of emergency.
- Try your best to prevent diarrhea and severe motion sickness that makes you vomit. If you know you are prone to seasickness, stay off cruise ships. If you go to Mexico or other countries where the food can be "iffy," carry a supply of antidiarrheal pills and do not drink the water, eat unpeeled fruits and vegetables, or eat any uncooked foods.
- If you are not a seasoned traveler and find yourself in a job where you will be taking frequent business trips, or if you de-

cide to take a major vacation, give yourself some practice before the big event. Start out with a day trip away from home, perhaps to a state park you've always wanted to see, or give yourself a day at the beach. Then go away for a whole weekend, stay at a hotel or inn, and eat all your meals in restaurants. Make notes of problem areas and devise creative ways to solve them.

- When you travel in a foreign country (and even in some remote areas of the United States), when you see a bathroom, use it. You never know when you'll find another one.
- Test your blood glucose about twice as often as you do at home. The stress of travel, changing time zones, and mixed-up eating times all have an effect on blood glucose, and you want to catch hyper- or hypoglycemia before is becomes a problem.

Relationships with Family and Friends

Your family and friends need to get used to the fact that you have diabetes. The disease has its greatest impact on you, but it also affects the people around you, especially those in your household.

You have a serious chronic disease and that's scary to those who love and care about you. Perhaps they're afraid you'll die soon (children are particularly prone to fearing the loss of a parent) or you'll go blind and won't be able to work and take care of them. Maybe the glucose monitor, bottles of pills, and vials of insulin freak them out. Maybe they're annoyed because right now all you think about is your eating plan and getting used to your various regimens, and you're paying less attention to them. Who knows what they are thinking. You won't know until you ask. If you want the support of your family and close friends, you need to talk things through with them. You need to tell them how you feel about having diabetes and find out how they feel about it. You need to tell them what scares you and find out what scares them.

It's up to you to initiate these conversations, and to some extent, it's up to you to educate the people close to you about your disease. It may be unfair if they don't take responsibility to learn about what affects you on their own, but it's up to you to get your needs met. There are a few enlightened partners who will go to the library or bookstore without being asked and read about diabetes, but for the most part, they will be the listeners, and you will be the expert.

For Penny, the worst part about having diabetes was her family. They were nice to her, but she felt as if they could have been more understanding about what she was going through.

Her children were in high school at the time she was diagnosed, and they hated having to sit down to supper when Penny needed to eat. It was too early for them, and they didn't realize that she had to eat. They didn't know anything about diabetes and they never bothered to learn. Her husband said that diabetes was just one more thing they have to get through.

Her kids are in college now, so it's just the two of them and their golden retriever at home. Her husband doesn't get home from work until at least 7:30, so she's learned to have a snack when she gets home at around 3:30. That way they can eat dinner together. The kids have gotten used to her eating habits, too. They know she gets cranky when she's really hungry and they say, "Oh, there goes Mom again." They don't pay much attention anymore.

Penny seems to have accepted the fact that whatever she wants her husband and children to know about diabetes, she will have to teach them, and she has gotten used to the fact that she will have to make all the compromises about food and eating. Since she is the family cook, she at least gets to control what's put on the table.

In the long run, taking the time to teach others about diabetes will be in your best interest. If people know what you can eat and what you can't, if they watch you test your blood glucose a few times and if they see how easy it is to give yourself an insulin injection, they will feel less strange around you and your diabetes. They also won't keep asking you the same questions over and over. "Are you sure you can eat this?" "Is this okay on your diet, hon?" "Now, tell me again: How many times a day do you have to use that machine?" This kind of nagging (and the feeling you get that the constant questions imply that they weren't paying attention in the first place) is extremely stress-producing, and over time, can place serious strain on a relationship.

If you are participating in diabetes classes or are a member of a support group, consider taking your family and maybe even some close friends along with you. This is one way for them to see a bunch of healthy-looking people who have diabetes, all of whom are taking it in stride, coping well and controlling their disease. It also goes a long way to demonstrate that your family is not the only one that this has happened to, and when they see how other spouses and children behave, they will have positive examples of good family functioning and caring support.

It's also a good idea to teach family members how to test blood glucose and give you an insulin injection. It's another opportunity for them to learn more about diabetes and how it is controlled, and it gives them a feeling of participation in your well-being. It also can come in handy in an emergency.

There are a number of ways in which family and friends can be a hindrance as well as a help and thus inadvertently sabotage your efforts to control your diabetes. This is highly stressful, and it is up to you to remedy the situation. But remember, you can never change other people's behavior, only your own. So in the following situations, it is up to you to decide how to react and what to do.

"Come on, one slice of pie isn't going to make any difference. It's not even that big a slice." If there are other people present, your only option here, at least for now, is to say, "No, thank you," or "No, I can't eat the pie." Repeat one of these responses until the message penetrates, and then later, when you have an opportunity to be alone, ask the person not to do that again. Say something like, "I know what I can eat, and it's not helpful to me when you coax me into doing something that will hurt me. Please don't do it anymore." If people persist, ask why they are being so hostile, and explain to them that urging you to harm yourself is a very angry, hostile reaction to your diabetes and to you.

Here's another stress-producing scenario: The minute you walk into someone's house and in front of all the other guests, the host says, "You can eat everything I made for dinner. I went out and bought a special cookbook just for this meal, and I made a really big effort to cook everything dietetic." Of course, you'll probably want to sink into the floor from embarrassment—and from the looks on the other guests' faces as they contemplate a meal of tasteless food. You have two choices here: The first is to say nothing; the second is to say, "Oh, thank you, but that really wasn't necessary. Diabetics can eat everything in moderation, just like everyone else." Then, when you get this person alone, you can explain how you felt and ask that it not be repeated.

9

Health Complications

Type I or Type II diabetes can result in some pretty severe complications over the years. However, the tighter you control your blood glucose, the less likely you are to suffer ill effects, and the less severe those effects will be.

If, after reading this chapter, you feel as though you have a problem, or are on the verge of one, see your physician right away. In general, warning signs of diabetic complications include: diminished or distorted vision; overwhelming, unexplained fatigue that doesn't go away; numbness, tingling, or loss of sensation anywhere in your body; chest pain; cuts or infections that take too long to heal; and constant headaches, which may be a sign of hypertension.

In older diabetics, complications progress more rapidly than in younger people. But if the elderly maintain good blood glucose control, they will have less nocturia (urination at night) and polyuria (frequent urination), two of the most irritating effects of diabetes. They also will suffer from fewer infections and their wounds will heal better and more quickly.

Treatments to Reduce Long-Term Complications

One of the most important sources of information about diabetes came from a recent ten-year study (1983-1993) conducted by the National Institute of Diabetes and Digestive and Kidney Diseases of the National Institutes of Health. Called the Diabetes Control and Complications Trial (DCCT), it studied the relationship between control of blood glucose and long-term complications of diabetes. Almost fifteen hundred volunteers with Type I diabetes participated in the randomized study. This means that half the study subjects followed conventional diabetes therapy (the control group) and half used intensive therapy: three or four daily insulin injections (or an insulin pump), testing blood glucose four to seven times a day, and adjusting insulin doses to food intake and exercise.

Results showed that diabetics who keep their blood glucose levels as close to normal as possible significantly lower their risk of complications. Specifically, it was not the dose of insulin that was the crucial factor, but rather keeping blood glucose normal (normal—not low). In other words, insulin is only a way to achieve the goal. The best way to do this is with intensive diabetes therapy.

The DCCT showed that by maintaining tight control, you can reduce your risk of eye disease by 76 percent, kidney disease by 50 percent, neuropathy by 60 percent, and cardiovascular disease by 50 percent. Unfortunately, these benefits were accompanied by a significantly increased incidence of severe hypoglycemia.

The Ongoing Veterans Affairs Cooperative Study on Glycemic Control and Complications has attempted to extend the DCCT by evaluating the effects of intensive insulin therapy in Type I diabetic men age forty to sixty-nine. The men succeeded in reducing their glycohemoglobin levels (the test that shows diabetes control over a three-month period) approximately two percentage points with little risk of severe hypoglycemia. Preliminary study results show that there has been no apparent effect on the incidence of cardiovascular disease.

Intensive Therapy

Intensive diabetes therapy (as opposed to conventional therapy, which you have read about in the first few chapters) is an attempt to imitate the way a normal pancreas responds to the body's need for insulin. It involves frequent blood glucose testing (four or five times a day) and consequent adjustment of insulin dose and meal plan depending on the results of the blood glucose test. In fact, the insulin dose and food intake may change from day to day.

If this seems like a bigger nuisance than conventional therapy, it is, but it works. Do not put yourself on intensive therapy, but you may want to discuss the possibility with your physician—who may have already broached the subject. If you do decide to try it, your physician or diabetes educator will show you how. It's somewhat complex although by no means impossible to learn.

Conventional diabetes therapy focuses on anticipating what you think your insulin needs will be for the next several hours, based on what you plan to eat. This assumes that you will be able to keep in balance all the factors that affect blood glucose. Sometime you can and sometimes you can't.

Intensive therapy assumes that your eating habits, physical activity, general health, and metabolism are not always the same. To help your body deal with these normal fluctuations, you must test your blood glucose frequently and then take a dose of insulin based both on what your future needs will be, as well as in response to your present blood glucose level. This attempts to mimic a normal pancreas, which is able to sense the level of glucose in the blood and then respond with a release of the correct amount of insulin.

People who usually derive the most benefit from intensive therapy are Type I diabetics who have had the disease for a while and who are adept at using conventional therapy. Diabetics in the early stages of Type I still have some functioning beta cells and therefore do not need intensive therapy.

Because the therapy requires so much attention, and because it causes the diabetes to always be "in your face," intensive therapy requires a high degree of commitment. But for people whose diabetes is in poor control, who are at especially high risk for complications, who are pregnant or who plan to become pregnant, or who have an unpredictable lifestyle, intensive therapy is worth it.

The DCCT was done on only Type I diabetics, but most diabetes specialists believe that it also can be beneficial for Type II diabetics. This makes sense because the focus of intensive therapy is on maintaining normal blood glucose, not on the type or amount of medication taken. In Type II, the goal is achieved mainly through diet and physical activity, although some Type II diabetics will require oral hypoglycemic agents, and maybe even insulin, to achieve tight control. Many diabetics, both Type I and Type II, say they feel better after they have been on intensive therapy for a while because their glucose-insulin patterns closely resemble normal ones.

The major goal of intensive therapy is precision: keeping blood glucose as close to normal as possible for as long as possible. However, this is not as uncomplicated as it sounds. First, there is the question: What precisely is normal? There is a normal *range,* but how do you decide which of a range of normal numbers is "normal enough"? Second, diabetics must decide how far they are willing to go in interrupting the flow of their daily life in order to achieve this tight control.

There is, as yet, no good answer to the first question, and the second decision is a function of your own values. How far out of your way are you willing to go in order to prevent complications? There is no "right" answer to this; it depends on your lifestyle, what your ultimate goals are, and how you see yourself in relation to your diabetes. Also, you don't have to make a decision this minute. The option to do intensive therapy will always be there should you decide to wait.

Having said all this, you should know that intensive therapy isn't for everyone. In fact, there are some people who probably should not begin intensive therapy: those who have a history of severe, frequent hypoglycemia; people younger than seven or older than seventy; cardiac patients; those with severe complications; people who cannot see well or who cannot manipulate diabetes equipment; those who abuse drugs or alcohol; and people who don't have the intellectual capacity to make reasonable decisions or who are otherwise unable to manage their own care.

> *But then there is Tom, who is mentally disabled and is on a modified form of intensive therapy—and who keeps his blood glucose in very tight control. He has had diabetes for more than fifty years (he was diagnosed with Type I when he was eighteen months old) and is so intellectually challenged that he has difficulty holding a conversation. Yet he tests his blood glucose eight times a day and follows a set schedule for insulin dosage. He takes a certain amount on the days he works a full day (he is a janitor in a high rise apartment building), another amount on days he works a half day, and another amount on days he doesn't work.*
>
> *Tom was put on this regimen by a physician some years ago, but now he avoids going to the doctor. He belongs to an HMO, and he feels he knows more about diabetes than his doc-*

tor. Because of his negative experiences with doctors over his lifetime, he doesn't want to have anything to do with them. Instead, he goes to a support group, led by a certified diabetes educator, and she tells him what to do and answers all of his questions.

Once in a while, however, he needs the services of a physician because of complications. He has had four laser treatments and one cataract removal operation. Tom knows that his eye problems arise from his diabetes, but he doesn't understand how. He has medals and certificates from the Eli Lilly Company and from the Joslin Clinic in Boston congratulating him on living with diabetes for fifty years.

For a person of such limited ability, Tom has been able to remain remarkably healthy for a long time with a serious disease. As long as he has a written schedule of when to test his blood glucose, how much insulin to take, and when and what to eat, he can do fine. He gets plenty of exercise at his job, so there's little to think about.

Insulin Infusion Pump

The insulin infusion pump is a major advance in diabetes therapy. This is a device about the size of a pager, worn outside the body, that pumps the required amount of insulin in a steady infusion into the body via tubing and a needle, which is usually changed every three days or so. It also can be commanded to send an extra surge of insulin, called a bolus, to compensate for a rise in blood glucose after eating. If you use a pump, you still have to test your blood glucose frequently and adjust your insulin dose as usual.

The advantage of a pump is that it provides a slow, constant flow of insulin, in addition to the bolus required to cover incoming food. Thus, using the pump more closely imitates the natural action of the pancreas. Because of the smoothness of the action of an insulin pump, most people feel better than they did on individual injections.

An external insulin pump sounds like a great idea—for people who are truly motivated and responsible. But there are some things to consider. First, it is part of a more complex system than what is involved in giving yourself individual injections. Therefore, you need to test your blood glucose more frequently, five or six times a day. Second, because the pump is a continuous infusion, you run a greater risk of developing hypoglycemia if you fail to keep careful track of your blood glucose. Third, some people develop a false sense of security with the pump. They believe that because the infusions are automatic, whatever they eat (and whatever exercise they stop doing) will be automatically covered by the pump. This is not true. You still have to follow your food plan and maintain your level of physical activity.

Fourth, an insulin pump takes a great deal of getting used to, calibrating doses and matching the need for a bolus to food intake. Fifth, the pump is expensive (up to $5,000), and you may have to go through a great deal of letter writing, cajoling, and threatening to get your health insurance company to pay for it; and even then, it might not. Medicare is an even tougher nut than a private insurance company when it comes to paying for medical devices.

Sixth, all kinds of things can go wrong and you may spend more time fiddling with the pump than you do giving yourself injections, especially when you are getting used to it. The tubing can get clogged or twisted (although use of Humulin BR and buffered velosulin human insulin have pretty much solved the problem of clogged tubing); if you place the needle in a poor site, it may fall out; the insulin can leak out around the infusion site and blood can get into the tubing; the battery runs down every now and then (but it will beep to let you know); and, like any automated equipment, it can stop working at an inconvenient time. However, as with all electronic devices, improvements will be made quickly and the price will fall. The pump is not for everyone, but it is one more way to make control of your diabetes easier and safer. And if you are willing to follow instructions and make sure it is operating correctly, the pump can be a great boon for insulin-dependent diabetics.

Long-Term Complications

Heart and Blood Vessel Problems

Diabetics are more likely than nondiabetics to develop heart and blood vessel (cardiovascular) diseases. No one knows exactly why this is so, but the best guess is that over time, high blood glucose damages vessels. In addition, diabetics tend to have higher blood fat and cholesterol, which is a primary risk factor for cardiovascular disease, especially the formation of blood clots, which cause heart attack and stroke.

The risk of cardiovascular disease in diabetics is compounded by being overweight (which increases the strain on the heart), having high blood pressure, and smoking. Major types of cardiovascular disease include:

- *Atherosclerosis.* Buildup of plaque deposits on the walls of vessels
- *Myocardial infarction.* Blockage of blood supply to the heart
- *Hypertension.* High blood pressure
- *Cardiovascular accident (stroke).* Blockage of blood supply to the brain
- *Peripheral vascular disease.* Pain in thigh or calf muscles when standing, walking, or exercising

Diabetic cardiovascular complications fall into two main categories: microangiopathy (small blood vessel disease) and macroangiopathy (large blood vessel disease). The former causes problems related to the eyes, kidneys, and, to some extent, the muscles of the heart.

Macroangiopathy has a major effect on the heart, but it also may cause damage to the brain and extremities. Blood vessels feeding the heart can become obstructed, resulting in pain (angina), partial blockage (heart attack), or complete blockage or rupture, which is usually fatal. If vessels leading to the brain are obstructed, the result is a stroke that causes the death of brain cells, which never regenerate. Depending on the location of the damage, the person may become unable to speak, think, or even breathe. Blockage in the legs is called peripheral vascular disease and can result in cramping pain when walking (intermittent claudication).

Macroangiopathy is treated in a variety of ways: angioplasty (reaming out a vessel to remove the blockage); laser surgery (to accomplish the same purpose); balloon angioplasty, in which a balloon is inserted into the vessel and inflated to squeeze the blockage against the wall of the vessel; and implantation of bypass grafts.

Nerve Problems

Neuropathy is disease or dysfunction of the nerves. Since you have nerves all over your body, any one or all of them can be damaged by poor blood glucose control. The mechanism of diabetic neuropathy is as follows: nerve tissue is surrounded by a protective sheath of cells called Schwann cells. These cells insulate the nerves, which you could think of as minute and highly sensitive electric wires. If excess blood glucose seeps into the Schwann cells, they will swell and put pressure on the nerves, which become irritated and often cause severe pain.

There are two types of neuropathy. Sensory neuropathy affects the sensory nerves that control the feeling in your body. Autonomic neuropathy affects nerves that control internal organs such as the kidneys, stomach, and intestines.

Depending on which nerves are affected, diabetics with sensory neuropathy often feel a tingling sensation, numbness, or coldness in their hands, arms, feet, and legs. Cold weather often worsens the condition. The extremities are the most common location for sensory neuropathy, which also is called peripheral neuropathy because it occurs at the outside (periphery) of your body. Symptoms are worse at night. Soon after going to bed, a person with diabetic neuropathy will experience a sensation of numbness, or a crawly or tingly sensation, and will have to get up and walk around. Sometimes the symptoms are worse: severe pain or complete absence of sensation, which means the nerves have died. Once a nerve has died, it will never grow back and the feeling in that site is lost forever.

In addition to pain and loss of feeling, sensory neuropathy creates other problems. For example, if you have lost sensation, you cannot feel when you have suffered a minor injury such as a blister or cut on your foot. Neither can you tell when your hands or feet have become dangerously cold, which can result in frostbite. And if you can't feel it, you may not realize it's there and will be unable to care for it. This can lead to infection and other more serious problems. Foot amputation is not uncommon in people who have serious diabetic sensory neuropathy. Moreover, muscles triggered by sensory nerves are no longer stimulated as they should be, which can lead to loss of muscle tone in affected areas. Muscles can shrink in size and bulk, which will impede your movement and gait in a variety of unpleasant ways.

Autonomic neuropathy affects nerves of the body that control involuntary processes such as respiration, digestion, kidney filtration, and blood circulation. Autonomic neuropathy is manifested in a number of ways and has a variety of symptoms and consequences:

- Nausea, vomiting, diarrhea, or constipation, which indicates that your gastrointestinal muscles have become less efficient
- Gastroparesis, the inability of the stomach to pass food into the small intestine as quickly as normal, which can cause blood glucose to go out of control because nutrients, including sugars, are absorbed from the small intestine
- Sudden drop in blood pressure when you stand up (orthostatic hypotension) or severely elevated blood pressure when you engage in physical activity
- Inability to discern when your bladder is full or trouble emptying the bladder completely because nerves that control bladder function have been damaged
- Trouble breathing or inappropriate heart rate (too fast or too slow for what you should expect)
- Sexual dysfunction of a wide variety of types (see chapter 11)

Although physicians can prescribe medication to ease many of the symptoms, they cannot restore lost nerve function. For the night "tinglies," diphenhydramine (Benadryl) often works. It can work during the day as well, but many people feel too drowsy to function, even on a very low dose. For lancinating or stabbing pains in the legs, phenytoin sodium (Dilantin) can help, as can amitriptyline hydrochloride (Elavil or Endep), nortriptyline hydrochloride (Aventyl or Pamelor), and imipramine hydrochloride (Tofranil or Janimine).

As with most health problems, the best defense is a good offense: prevent neuropathy by keeping blood glucose normal. Also, pay special attention to personal hygiene, such as foot and skin care (see chapter 7).

People with diabetic neuropathy should not drink alcohol—not even in moderation. Even cough syrup or other medicine that contains alcohol must be avoided. It will only worsen the condition.

Eye Problems

The eyes are incredibly vulnerable to the effects of high blood glucose, the most serious of which is diabetic retinopathy. The retina is a thin, light-sensitive membrane at the back of the eye. Retinopathy (disease or dysfunction of the retina) is caused when high levels of blood glucose damage the blood vessels that supply the retina. Most people who have had diabetes for more than twenty-five or thirty years will have at least minor damage to these vessels, but few people go blind now because with high-tech diagnostic and treatment methods, the disease can be treated in its early stages. This is why it is absolutely crucial for you to have a dilated eye examination at least once a year. Most people who have early diabetic retinopathy don't realize it.

Diabetic retinopathy has two stages: the early, nonproliferative stage (also called background retinopathy) and proliferative retinopathy. In the early stage, damaged blood vessels leak into the retina causing it to swell. When the fluid collects in the central part of the retina, this, too, swells (macular edema) and blurs vision. Macular edema can be treated by laser surgery.

During the later, more serious stage, new and abnormal blood vessels grow over the surface of the retina. They may rupture and bleed into the clear gel that fills the center of the eyeball (vitreous humor). This blocks passage of light through the eyeball so it cannot reach the retina at the back. If light cannot get through, vision dims. If the process continues unchecked, blindness will occur. If a serious hemorrhage occurs, vision will be lost. Laser surgery, however, can remove blood from the eye, thus successfully restoring vision.

Another problem is that blood vessels leaking into the retina can cause scar tissue on the retina, which pulls it into a distorted shape, and eventually it can detach from the back of the eye. Detached retina can be treated with laser surgery, but the restored vision will not be perfect.

Cataracts and glaucoma occur in nondiabetics as well as diabetics, although the latter are at increased risk. A cataract is a condition in which the lens of the eye grows cloudy and opaque, thus diminishing the amount of light that reaches the eyeball and retina. Treatment consists of removing the diseased lens and replacing it with an artificial one, thus restoring vision—often better than it was before.

Glaucoma is caused by increased pressure in the eyeball, and everyone over age forty, diabetic or not, is at risk for this condition, which is one of the leading causes of blindness. Glaucoma is detected by measuring eyeball pressure, a routine part of an eye examination. It can be successfully treated with eye drops that correct fluid pressure.

If these eye problems sound scary, they are. There are, however, steps you can take to minimize your risk of diabetic eye problems:

- Most importantly, keep your blood glucose levels in tight control.
- When you are first diagnosed with diabetes, inform your ophthalmologist and make certain that you have a dilated eye examination (where the physician puts drops in your eyes to visualize the retina, blood vessels, and all other structures) at least once a year.
- If you notice any changes in vision, no matter how slight, go to the eye doctor (a physician, not an optometrist) immediately. If the trouble is a diabetic eye problem, it is best to diagnose and treat it early.

Kidney Problems

Diabetic nephropathy, or disease of the kidneys, is caused by a mechanism similar to that of diabetic retinopathy: damage to blood vessels and nephrons as a result of long-term high blood glucose. Kidney damage is particularly serious because you cannot live without them, and for diabetics, damage to one kidney usually implies present or highly potential damage to both.

The kidneys are highly vascular organs; that is, they contain many blood vessels, which serve as adjuncts to the nephrons, which are the main filtering units of the kidneys. Nephrons filter out waste products carried to them by the bloodstream. The cleaned blood recirculates once it has dumped its load of waste into the nephrons. Waste is then transported to larger tubules and then to the outside of the body in the form of urine. Therefore, if the blood vessels of the kidney or the nephrons are damaged, toxic waste cannot be removed and it builds up in the bloodstream and will eventually kill you.

Diabetic nephropathy can be prevented, but it cannot be reversed once the process has started. If the problem gets so bad that you reach a point called end-stage renal disease (renal is a medical term for kidney function), you would need dialysis (an artificial method of removing toxins from the blood) and a kidney transplant. If, at the time you need one, there is a lot of competition for a kidney (and there always is), diabetics and people with some other chronic diseases are put at the bottom of the list.

Symptoms of diabetic nephropathy, which start so gradually that you hardly notice them and then increase in intensity, include swelling of the ankles, hands, and face; loss of appetite; a metallic taste in the mouth; skin irritation due to "sweating out" some toxins that should be excreted in urine; difficulty managing blood glucose; and fatigue. If you notice any of these symptoms, call your physician right away.

Kidney damage is one of the worst things that can happen to a diabetic. Even if you don't die of it, treatment of end-stage renal disease is a ghastly procedure involving uncomfortable sessions of dialysis four or five times a week, either at home or in a hospital outpatient department.

It is much smarter to prevent kidney disease than to have to treat it. Here are some ways to do that:

- Keep your blood glucose in tight control.
- Keep your blood pressure normal: no higher than 140/90. High blood pressure stresses the kidneys, but there is a variety of medications to keep it in check if necessary.
- Treat all urinary tract infections, no matter how minor. Symptoms include cloudy or bloody urine, frequent urination, pain or burning when urinating, and the feeling of always needing to urinate.
- Have a routine urinalysis at least once a year. The test includes the following elements that indicate potential kidney dysfunction: protein in the urine (if yours shows a spillage of protein, eat less meat and poultry); micoalbuminurea, an indication of early problems; and creatinine, which shows the presence of certain waste products that should be excreted by the kidneys.

Hyperglycemia

You have hyperglycemia when your blood glucose is 180 mg/dl or higher, when measured at the same time of day, for three or more days in a row. However, there are times when this may happen and you are not "officially" considered hyperglycemic, such as when you have a temporary illness or when your physician readjusts your insulin dose.

The most frequent cause of high blood glucose is too much food. If you eat more than your food plan calls for, your exercise regimen and diabetes medication will not be able to handle the excess and you will become hyperglycemic. A secondary cause is not getting enough exercise.

Hyperglycemia often does not result in physical symptoms, but some people experience some of the same things they did right before their initial diagnosis: thirst, fatigue, or blurry vision. With or without symptoms, the only way to diagnose hyperglycemia is by blood glucose monitoring.

If you become hyperglycemic and before you call your physician, there are some things you can do yourself to lower your blood glucose, for instance:

- If you have made mistakes in the timing or dosage of insulin injections, correct them.
- If you have gained weight recently, lose it.
- If you are using a new oral hypoglycemic agent or are taking another medication temporarily, the hyperglycemia may disappear when you get used to the new agent or when you finish the other drug.
- Test your blood glucose at the same times every day to avoid natural fluctuations that you may have mistakenly believed was hyperglycemia.
- Adjust your insulin dose for such an eventuality, but only as you have been instructed. Do not "experiment" with dosages on your own.

If none of these things works and you remain hyperglycemic, notify your physician, who will probably ask you to come into the office for more sophisticated blood tests, and in the meantime, may adjust the dosage of your oral hypoglycemic agent or insulin. Depending on the results of the blood tests, if you have not been taking insulin you mady have to begin.

Diabetic Ketoacidosis

If blood sugar gets so high that your body starts burning fat stores for energy, you may start producing ketone bodies which build up and spill over into the urine. The combination of high blood glucose, ketone bodies, dehydration, and various chemical imbalances, if untreated, leads to a condition known as ketoacidosis, most commonly seen in Type I diabetics, although it is not unknown in Type II diabetics.

Ketoacidosis is a serious medical emergency. Symptoms include nausea, stomach pain, vomiting, chest pain, rapid and shallow breathing, and difficulty staying awake. If you have these signs, get to an emergency room right away because ketoacidosis can kill you. It develops gradually, however. If you have been testing your blood glucose on schedule and if you have educated yourself about diabetes, you will be able to see it coming and can thus do something to prevent it.

When you have another illness on top of your diabetes, you are at higher risk for ketoacidosis; therefore it is vital to check your blood glucose frequently. Also, when you are home sick, you should ask someone to check on you a few times a day. Ask your spouse or a friend (someone close who has a key to your house) to call, and instruct them that, if you don't answer the phone, they should go to your house; if they find you unconscious, they should call an ambulance without delay.

Diabetic ketoacidosis is treated with intravenous fluids to dilute the blood glucose and rehydrate you. Chemicals (most often potassium and sodium) are added to the intravenous fluid to correct the body's imbalances, and insulin is given to get glucose out of the bloodstream and into the cells. Once blood glucose levels have dropped to an acceptable level, the body needs fuel so it will not manufacture more ketones, so glucose is added to the intravenous solution. Emergency room physicians will get you stabilized and then will admit you to the hospital where you will stay for a day or two to make certain that you have safely passed the crisis.

Matthew got either the stomach flu or food poisoning and started vomiting. He couldn't eat. He knew enough not to take as much insulin as usual, but other than that he didn't think too much about it.

After three days he felt better and went back to school, but on the fourth day he felt awful. He was in glee club practice and had to leave the room to throw up. He got sent home from school and his mother called the doctor, who instructed her to take Matthew right to the emergency room. When he got there, they took some blood and started intravenous fluids because he was dehydrated. He had to wait about two hours for the blood tests to come back, and when they did, Matthew was admitted to the intensive care unit. He was so dehydrated that he got eight liters (about eight quarts) of fluid before he had to urinate.

Hypoglycemia

Most of the diabetics who suffer occasional bouts of hypoglycemia are those who take insulin. It is rarer, but not unknown, in people who take oral hypoglycemic agents.

You have low blood glucose (hypoglycemia) if it measures less than 60 mg/dl. Many times you will know that your blood sugar is low by the way you feel (shakiness, nervousness, dizziness, weakness, irritability, hunger, pounding heart), but never depend on that. Always test it, because some of the symptoms are the same as those of illnesses unrelated to diabetes and others are the same as hyperglycemia.

If you are hypoglycemic, do something about it right away because the problem can escalate rapidly, and could lead to convulsions or unconsciousness. Both of these consequences of untreated hypoglycemia are extremely serious, and if you are alone, they are life threatening.

Hypoglycemia is usually caused by not eating when you should. Any time you skip a meal or delay it for a while, you risk hypoglycemia because you have too little glucose in your bloodstream for the amount of insulin circulating there. The insulin acts on what little sugar is available to it, and because you don't replenish the supply, your blood glucose level dips drastically.

A secondary cause is exercising more than you usually do without eating enough to compensate for the increased physical activity. The more you exercise, the lower your blood glucose will drop, and if you are taking insulin, you compound the problem.

One cause of low blood glucose is losing a great deal of weight without seeing your physician and having the dosage of insulin or oral hypoglycemics adjusted, and another cause is taking too much insulin. This last condition is also called insulin reaction or insulin shock.

The DCCT showed that the more tightly diabetics tried to control their disease, the more likely they were to have hypoglycemia and insulin reaction, which once again points to the importance of testing blood glucose frequently. A rule of thumb is: The harder you try to achieve tight control, the more often you should test your blood.

Some Type I diabetics have low blood glucose at night (nocturnal hypoglycemia). For this reason, you should not increase your dose of intermediate-acting insulin before supper or bedtime without first testing your blood glucose to make certain it is not low. If you have nocturnal hypoglycemia, it may wake you up or you may have a headache in the morning. If you are awakened, test your blood sugar and take corrective action if it is too low.

By morning, it may have corrected itself naturally, and your blood glucose may even be a little high. This is called rebound (Somogyi effect) and is your body's response to abnormally low blood glucose. Rebound can take several hours, during which sugar stored in the liver is released into the bloodstream and may elevate your blood glucose to as high as 250 to 300 for twelve to twenty-four hours. Eventually, the condition will resolve itself, as the extra sugar is used by the cells or returns to the liver for storage. If you try to compensate by taking extra insulin or exercising more vigorously than usual, you're likely to make things worse, and your blood sugar could swing down precipitously. If you experience rebound, the best thing to do is to eat and exercise normally and take your usual dose of insulin. If things don't even out in three days, call your physician.

General guidelines for treating low blood glucose include:

- Treat it immediately in order to prevent more serious problems.
- Carry a supply of carbohydrates (for example, fat-free hard candy, but not chocolate) with you at all times in case of sudden hypoglycemia. This is particularly important when you are exercising or driving a car on a long trip.
- Don't panic. Insulin reaction can be frightening, but if you treat it immediately, it will pass. Eat some rapidly absorbed, high-carbohydrate food; sit or lie down; and wait ten or fifteen minutes for it to reach your bloodstream. If your next scheduled meal isn't for an hour or more, have a low-fat snack. If you don't feel much better in another fifteen minutes or so, call your physician.
- Always carry identification in case things get out of control. The ID should clearly state that you are a diabetic, and it should include your name, address, and phone number; your physician's phone number; and someone to call in an emergency.
- Follow your physician's recommended insulin dosage schedule in the event of weight loss.
- Alcohol causes low blood sugar. Follow the suggested guidelines for alcohol and food in chapter 3.

- Make certain your physician knows about all medications you are taking, even the over-the-counter drugs. Some may put you at increased risk of hypoglycemia.

It is unlikely that you will fall unconscious or have a convulsion, but if you do, you need medical attention immediately. You should receive an injection of a hormone called glucagon, which is produced in the pancreas and raises blood glucose by stimulating the liver to release its stored sugar.

Anyone can give you a shot of glucagon; therefore your close friends, a trusted work colleague, and family should be taught how to do it. If no such person is around, you should be taken to a hospital by ambulance.

Glucagon takes five to ten minutes to work (you should be placed on your side in case you vomit), that is, until the convulsions stop and you regain consciousness. Once you feel better, eat a low-fat, high-carbohydrate, high-protein snack.

If the first injection doesn't bring you around, you should be given another, and if that doesn't work, you need to be rushed to an emergency room, where you will probably get an intravenous injection of glucagon.

Your physician will give you a prescription for a glucagon kit, which contains a bottle of the hormone in powder form and a syringe prefilled with solution to dilute it, and you should keep it with you at all times. When the expiration date arrives, throw it out and get a new one.

The following is the emergency treatment for hypoglycemia (one of any of the following):

- Three glucose tablets
- A half cup of fruit juice
- A half cup of regular soft drink (not diet)
- One cup of skim milk
- Six or seven hard candies (with sugar)
- Five sugar cubes
- Ten jelly beans
- One tablespoon of honey
- A small tube of cake frosting

Infections

Diabetics are more prone to infections than are nondiabetics. Infections in diabetics often take longer to heal because excess blood glucose can interfere with immune system function. White blood cells—the heart of the immune system—attack and kill invading viruses, bacteria, and fungi, but if these cells are not operating at peak efficiency because they are hampered by excessive glucose, the invading microorganisms get the upper hand and you get an infection. To complicate things, the invading germs feed on the excess glucose and multiply.

Other complications of diabetes tend to increase your risk of infection and make the ones that you do get harder to cure. For example, if you have bladder neuropathy and can't empty it completely, a little urine sits in your bladder and provides a breeding ground for microorganisms. Or if you have peripheral neuropathy, you are less likely to be aware of little cuts and scrapes, thus leaving them open to infection.

If you get an infection—of any type and anywhere on your body—see your physician, who will prescribe an appropriate antibiotic, antiviral, or antifungal medication. When you fill the prescription, take all of it. Many antibiotics relieve symptoms quickly, sometimes within a few hours, but this does not mean that the microorganism has been killed. So no matter how good you feel, finish the pills.

Diabetes and Minor Illnesses

Everyone gets colds and the flu. Most people fall victim to food poisoning once or twice. Few people fail to stay away from the surgeon's knife or the dentist's pliers for their entire lives, and there's hardly anyone who has never spent a night as a hospital patient or a few hours in an emergency room.

For nondiabetics, colds and the flu are generally taken in stride (and there's even some pleasure in snuggling under the covers with a good book and a supply of orange juice and hot tea while co-workers are slaving away in the office), and as soon as the unpleasantness of the illness is over, they forget it.

For diabetics, these minor illnesses require a bit more attention. Diabetics can certainly get through them all right, but they have to pay attention to things other than making sure they have enough tissues and cough syrup on hand. Once again, blood glucose must be monitored especially carefully during physical illness.

Any illness, no matter how minor or how quickly it is resolved, puts stress on the body, and stress causes certain hormonal changes, which in turn causes the liver to increase its production of glucose. The liver also releases stored glucose into the bloodstream to deal with the stress of illness.

At the same time, some of the hormonal changes make cells more resistant to insulin, which means that circulating glucose will not be as easily absorbed into the cells. So you have a double whammy: increased circulating glucose and increased release of glucose from the liver. This creates a potential for danger, which is why you need to be especially vigilant about your blood glucose, as well as ketones in the urine if you take insulin.

Although you must follow your physician's instructions for treating the underlying illness and take the medications prescribed, you should also follow a number of general guidelines for managing your diabetes while you are ill:

- Drink sufficient liquids in order to prevent dehydration. If your blood glucose is higher than usual and spills over into your urine, the excess tends to draw additional water from your cells causing unusually large volumes of urine. Therefore, you need to compensate for this loss by drinking at least eight ounces of fluid (water, diet soda, bouillon) every hour.
- You may lose your appetite, but by now you know how important it is to follow your meal plan, so even though you don't feel like eating, do it anyway. (If you absolutely can't eat, or if you are vomiting a lot, you must call your physician.) Eat foods that are bland (chicken, gelatin, rice, whole grain cereal with skim milk, plain broiled or grilled meat, light vegetables) and alternate them with soups and other nourishing liquids. It is particularly important to eat your usual amount of carbohydrate-containing foods.
- Always take your full dose of diabetes medication unless you are instructed otherwise by your physician. Don't skip doses, even if you don't feel like eating.
- Monitor your blood glucose every three or four hours—night and day. It's a nuisance to set your alarm to wake up in the middle of the night, but do it anyway. It's not forever. If your

blood glucose is too high or too low, follow the guidelines above for hyper- and hypoglycemia.

- Keep your medicine cabinet well stocked with things like cough and cold medicines (note the warning about ephedrine in chapter 5 in the section "Cough and Cold Medicines"), antidiarrheal pills, laxatives, aspirin or acetaminophen, and the like so you don't have to go to the drugstore when you fall ill.
- Keep a bottle of regular insulin on hand even if you don't usually use it, because if you need extra insulin when you are sick, this is the type you will be told to take.
- Do not exercise until you are better, because it can have a paradoxic effect and elevate your blood glucose.

Diabetes and Surgery

As soon as you find out you need surgery, you will see a surgeon for a preoperative visit. The first thing you need to tell the surgeon is that you are a diabetic. Even if your physician says it's a minor procedure, speak up. (There's an old saw that says that minor surgery is what happens to someone else; yours is always major.)

Surgery is one of the most stressful things your body (and you) will ever have to endure, and by now, you know what stress does to your blood glucose. If you are a candidate for emergency surgery, speak up immediately when you are admitted to the emergency room. Whatever is wrong with you will already have affected your blood glucose and it needs to be brought under control right away. If you are unconscious, you have to hope for the best. This is a major reason why you need to carry or wear identification as a diabetic, as well as a strong reason to tell close friends, who should mention your diabetes if they accompany you to the hospital.

In addition to telling your surgeon, when you enter the hospital, make certain the admitting nurse and all the nurses on the unit know that you are a diabetic. You don't need to bring your own blood glucose monitor to the hospital because one will be supplied for you. If your blood testing routine is different from what the nurses have planned for you, tell them how often you usually monitor your blood.

Request a consultation with the hospital dietician and mention what you like and what you don't like to eat. Hospital food is notoriously awful (the same companies cater to hospitals as to airlines and prisons), and a diabetic diet can be even worse. If you speak to the dietician, you may have a chance of getting something palatable to eat, but even that's not a sure thing.

But there's no reason why you have to exist entirely on hospital food. Your family and friends can bring you packages of goodies and many restaurants will deliver to hospitals. I had a cerebral hemorrhage a few years ago (before I became diabetic) and spent a week in neurosurgical intensive care. When I finally felt like eating again, my friend Janis brought me delicious lasagna, which the nurses let me keep in their refrigerator, and twice another patient and I shared Chinese take-out. In between times, I ate out of the fruit basket brought by another friend and devoured all the candy that came my way. Except for the candy and the excess cheese in the lasagna, it was a fine diabetic diet—supplemented by overcooked broccoli, tasteless chicken, and applesauce supplied by the hospital.

During surgery, your blood glucose will be constantly monitored. If you have been taking oral hypoglycemic agents, you may be asked to discontinue them for a day or so before the operation and you may be given insulin during the procedure. It all depends on how stable your blood glucose is, the type of medication you take, and the past experience of the surgeon.

The postoperative goal is to stabilize your blood glucose as quickly as possible for two major reasons. Elevated blood glucose decreases the number of fibroblasts in the blood. These cells help in wound healing. High blood glucose also retards production of white blood cells, which prevent and fight infection.

When you come home from the hospital following surgery, you need to test your glucose more frequently than usual, probably twice as often. In addition, you may need professional help with your eating plan if your appetite is still a little shaky. In fact, if you know you are going to have surgery, you should make an appointment with your diabetes educator to devise a postoperative meal plan.

10

Societal Issues

Health Insurance

You absolutely must have health insurance. If you work, you will probably buy it as part of your employer's benefit package. If your employer does not provide it, if you are self-employed, or if you are ineligible to be a dependent of your spouse's policy (or if you don't have a spouse), buy a policy yourself. Yes, it's expensive, but so are your car payments and a home mortgage, and you consider those an absolutely necessity of life. Health insurance is equally essential.

As a private person, you have two main choices about how you buy health insurance. You can either go it alone and buy an individual policy, or you can join an organization and become eligible for its group health benefits. Both have advantages and disadvantages, and you will have to do research to find out which is the best and most economical way to go.

Before you are issued a policy, you will be given a form to fill out about your general health and past medical history. When you come to the check-off box about diabetes, don't lie. If you do, you will never be able to present a claim for health care that has anything remotely to do with the disease. Or if you do present a claim, the carrier will find out you lied (and it *will* find out) and punish you. The two most common forms of punitive action are refusing to pay any diabetes-related claims and cancellation of your policy.

Whichever way you purchase health insurance, and whichever type you buy, you will receive a contract. Read it carefully—even the fine print—because you have a chronic disease and a preexisting condition, so you may be in for a rude surprise when filing claims for diabetes-related expenses. There are some important things diabetics need to know before making a decision about purchasing health insurance:

- Are there limits on the number of times you can visit your primary care physician each year?
- Does the plan reimburse for diabetes education or services of a nutritionist, exercise therapist, and other nonmedical specialists?
- Are diabetes supplies (syringes, glucose monitors, lancets, test strips, and the like) covered?
- What about prescriptions: is there a plan to reduce costs? If so, are there restrictions on the types of drugs covered, such as generic only? Will you have a copayment, and how many times can a prescription be refilled?
- Are medical specialist services covered, and are there restrictions such as a requirement for referral from a primary care physician (called a gatekeeper in many managed care plans)?
- Are there restrictions on what hospitals you can use?
- Are you covered when you are out of the country?

Major Types

Fee-for-service insurance, sometimes called traditional or conventional plan health insurance, is based on the payment of a premium (either directly to the insurance carrier or indirectly through an employer) in exchange for which some portion of health care expenses is reimbursed. The size of the portion and the type of expenses reimbursed vary widely depending on the plan purchased, which of course varies with the premium price. In a fee-for-service plan, the provider (physician, hospital, or other health provider) first bills the insurance company and then bills the patient for whatever is not covered. The latter is called balance billing. You can negotiate this sum with your physician.

Health maintenance organizations (HMOs) are managed care insurance plans that an individual or family joins as a dues-paying member for a flat monthly or quarterly fee (which tends to rise as the organization's expenses increase). The member receives almost all health care at little or no additional cost. Most HMOs charge a small per-visit fee in order to discourage unnecessary trips to the doctor; this practice will likely become more common in the future, and the per-visit fee will rise.

A preferred provider organization (PPO) is another type of controlled managed care plan. In this arrangement, physicians and other health care providers arrange with an insurer to discount their fees. Providers are then paid by the insurer, with patients paying a small per-visit fee. If you are a member of a PPO, you receive full coverage if you choose a physician from the preferred list. If you choose an "outside" physician, you will pay most of the bill yourself. You also may be penalized by losing future benefits.

Medicare is a federal program, enacted by an amendment to the Social Security Act, that provides hospital and medical care coverage for people age sixty-five and older, as well as for some individuals who have been disabled for more than twenty-four months. Medicare is not charity, any more than are Social Security benefits. It is a government entitlement program that is designed to cover very basic health care services, such as hospitalization, skilled nursing, diagnostic tests, emergency care, and some durable medical equipment such as wheelchairs, walkers, and crutches. More than three million Medicare recipients have diabetes.

Medicaid is a joint federal-state program, also created by the Social Security Act, that provides health services to people who live at or below the federal poverty level and have no other way to pay for health care. Eligibility requirements and services provided vary from state to state.

Using COBRA When Changing Jobs

COBRA stands for Consolidated Omnibus Budget Reconciliation Act. COBRA is a federal law that protects you when you leave your job, whether you quit or were fired, so that for eighteen months or until you find another job with health insurance benefits, you may participate with full coverage in the health insurance plan of the job you left. You will have to pay the premiums yourself, and the carrier (health insurance company) may charge you up to 2 percent more than it charges the employer, but this is always cheaper than buying an individual policy.

Once you leave your job, you have sixty days to sign up for COBRA benefits, but the best thing is to do it right away. Even if you are moving on to another job immediately, take the COBRA benefits because there may be a waiting period of one to six months before you are eligible for health insurance benefits on your new job. Even if you are eligible right away, what if you fall and break your leg over the weekend between the old job and the new one?

If you are disabled, your COBRA coverage can be extended to twenty-nine months, but you may not be able to make a case that diabetes alone (with no disabling complications) constitutes a disability.

If after eighteen months you have not found a job, you may be eligible for something called a conversion policy. This means that when your COBRA coverage runs out, the carrier will offer to cover you on the same policy—at a much larger premium, of course. About thirty-five states require insurers to offer conversion policies. When the offer is made, you have thirty days to respond.

Managed Care

Managed care is the most rapidly growing segment of the health care payment system in the United States. HMOs are the purest form of managed care, although all health insurance plans now use some type of managed care system. More than sixty million Americans are enrolled in HMOs, and 95 percent of employee health care benefits are under some type of managed care. In addition, Medicare and Medicaid are moving toward managed care payment systems. About 3.5 million Medicare beneficiaries and eight million Medicaid recipients are enrolled in managed care programs.

Although managed care is a complex system of paying for health care, a good brief definition is: an arrangement whereby someone is interposed between patients and health care providers. This someone has the authority to place restrictions on how and from whom patients may receive services and what services are to be provided in any given situation.

Moreover, this someone is not your health professional; it is usually an employee of an insurance company or health maintenance organization. In very broad strokes, here's how it works: You go to your physician, who makes a decision about the type of health care you require. But that decision is not final; unless it is an emergency, your health insurance company will have to approve what the physician wants to do.

In reality, things aren't quite this bad. Physicians don't have to make a phone call for every little thing they do because insurance companies have devised lists of what they believe are appropriate procedures and treatments for various ailments. These are the things for which the insurance carrier will reimburse you or your physician or other health care provider. For out of the ordinary procedures or treatments, you will need to obtain approval from your carrier. It's a nuisance and that's why so many physicians and patients don't like managed care.

However, managed care was instituted for a reason, and it has had some positive fallout for both physicians and patients, diabetics in particular. Health care costs in the United States have been escalating beyond all reason, far outstripping all rates of inflation. In addition, there are about forty-five million Americans who have no health insurance at all (not even Medicare and Medicaid) and who have to pay for everything out of their own pockets—or go without care.

Total health care expenditures for diabetics amount to about 14.6 percent of all health care expenditures in the United States. Total direct cost of the diabetes component of health care is about $50 billion, and the indirect cost from lost productivity caused by complications and death is another $50 billion. That's big, big bucks—for society in general as well as for diabetic individuals.

One of the reasons why health care costs so much is that so many physicians prescribe inappropriate and unnecessary procedures and treatments. They do this for two major reasons: plain old greed and a perceived need to practice "defensive medicine." The first motivation needs no explanation, but you may not know what defensive medicine is. The incidence of medical malpractice lawsuits has escalated so dramatically in the past few decades that physicians are perpetually terrified of being sued, so they perform every diagnostic test and procedure they can think of in an effort to cover all bases and to prove to the plaintiff's lawyers that they did everything reasonable and possible in the care of the patient suing.

Medical malpractice suits, both reasonable and frivolous, have reached epidemic proportions, and health insurance companies had to foot the bill to pay for these defensive (and usually medically unnecessary) procedures. They have no way to control who sues a physician, but they do have control over what they will or will not reimburse. So they started clamping down and instituting much more stringent reimbursement policies.

If your physician says you have to come to the office three or four times a year for a diabetes checkup, and you must have a variety of blood tests and medications, your carrier will reimburse with no questions asked because that is standard care for diabetes. But if your physicians wants you to have a stress test in the absence of cardiac symptoms or a brain scan when you have not complained of anything wrong with your head, the carrier will say, "No way!" Those tests would be unnecessary and inappropriate.

Insurers manage health care costs in four general ways. First, physicians and other providers are given financial incentives to use fewer services and to discourage patients from overusing services. For diabetics, this means that your primary care physician might discourage you from seeing an endocrinologist or flat-out refuse to provide a referral. Second, managed care organizations designate certain providers who will give necessary care at the least cost; the practice patterns of these providers are closely monitored by the organization, especially the number of referrals to specialists. Third, insurance policies control and limit the services for which a managed care organization will pay. This means that if you want to see a podiatrist or nutritionist, for example, you may not be reimbursed. Fourth, various mechanisms discourage enrollment of high-risk patients: those with preexisting conditions such as diabetes. Care of people with diabetes costs three times as much as nondiabetics; therefore, many insurers will try their hardest to keep diabetics off their rolls and will use a variety of unethical and illegal tactics to do so.

Some other ways in which managed care companies oversee health care costs include:

- Except in emergencies, requiring approval before a patient is admitted to a hospital
- Conducting an ongoing review of patients' treatments
- Day-to-day management of cases that require long-term and/or expensive care
- Review of discharged hospital patients' medical records to determine the quality and necessity of all procedures and other elements of care

American consumers of health care have benefited by not being subjected to unnecessary tests and treatments. All procedures carry risk and often have serious side effects. The less you are exposed to unnecessary risk, the better off you are, and this way you do not have to pay for something you didn't need in the first place.

Most physicians hate managed care. First, managed care reduces the number of medical procedures they perform because carriers will pay for only those they deem necessary, and this reduces the income of doctors since medical procedures are their most profitable source of income. Second, physicians do not like having to ask permission to provide the treatments for which they have been trained. Most physicians with busy practices have had to hire people who do nothing all day long but deal with insurance companies. This is expensive.

Managed care is generally unpleasant, but will be good for American society in the long run. Anything that brings down the cost of providing health care, but doesn't lower the quality of that care, is desirable. The problem is determining whether managed care organizations (that is, every health insurance carrier in the country) have taken so many cost-cutting steps that they have indeed jeopardized quality of care in some instances.

Little research has been done on the effects of managed care on diabetics. Payment incentives have encouraged routine initiation of insulin therapy on an outpatient basis, which is a benefit, but the incentives probably have negatively affected the way some hospitalized diabetics with complications have been treated. Managed care organizations are inconsistent in their policies regarding reimbursement for diabetes education, self-management training, nutrition counseling, self blood glucose monitors, and test strips (several states now mandate coverage of monitors and strips). Coverage for the complications of diabetes is generally excellent.

In addition, although most internists can provide good diabetic care and many diabetics do not need the services of a specialist, some primary care physicians do not know as much about diabetes as they ought to. However, no studies have been done to compare the quality of diabetes care between primary care physicians and specialists.

Federal Spending

The U.S. General Accounting Office recently studied Medicare claims of people with diabetes. In early 1997, it released its report: 168,000 people made such claims in 1994. The report also noted that, despite the importance of education and preventive care, most Medicare beneficiaries do not receive recommended education and monitoring services.

For instance, while more than 90 percent of the fee-for-service beneficiaries saw their physicians at least twice that year, only 40 percent had an eye examination, and only about 20 percent received glycohemoglobin tests. The figures were similar for Medicare beneficiaries in HMOs.

In addition, the report noted that people with diabetes use more health care services than those who do not—they have two to three times as many contacts with physicians and emergency rooms, two to three times more hospital outpatient visits, and three times more hospitalizations. They also are three times more likely to live in a nursing home.

Partly as a result of the GAO report and partly in reaction to Congressional pressure, in the summer of 1997, President Clinton signed the balanced budget agreement that carried a large boost in funding for diabetes research and control. First, Medicare benefits were increased by $2.1 billion for people with diabetes. Second, the agreement provided for a five-year payout of $150 million for research into juvenile diabetes and another $150 million to pay for prevention and treatment of diabetes among American Indians, who suffer from diabetes at more than three times the rate of other population groups.

Employment

Job Discrimination

Legally, you cannot be discriminated against because you have diabetes. Legally, you cannot be discriminated against because of your gender or religion. But legal restrictions have about as much to do with the real world of discrimination as lemon meringue pie has to do with building the Empire State Building. Sooner or later, if it hasn't happened already, you will be the victim of some form of discrimination on the job because you have diabetes. Therefore, the issue isn't whether it will happen but rather how you will handle it.

Insulin-dependent people with diabetes are barred from employment in several areas: the military (more about this later), field positions in federal and local law enforcement agencies, positions aboard ships where captaincy may be required, piloting private and commercial aircraft, and working on federal contracts that require certain types of travel, as well as air traffic control, and truck, bus, and ambulance driving. Some of these restrictions have been instituted because of fear that has no basis in reality, but certain occupations in which an episode of severe hypoglycemia could endanger lives carry justified limitations.

A number of attempts have been made to fight back against unwarranted discrimination. One of the most famous was *Joel R. Davis* v. *Edwin Meese III.* Davis, an otherwise qualified applicant with insulin-dependent diabetes, was turned down for a position as an FBI special agent. He sued the agency, but the United States District Court found that the FBI's policy of excluding diabetics on insulin did not violate the law because, according to the Court, the FBI "could not provide reasonable accommodation to insulin-dependent diabetics by permanently assigning them to limited duties or refraining from sending them on assignments that would substantially increase the risk of a severe hypoglycemic occurrence without deteriorating the services provided to the public and compromising the functions of the FBI." This ruling has served as a precedent for several other federal lawsuits by pilots, interstate truck drivers, and air traffic controllers.

The Federal Rehabilitation Act (FRA) of 1973 and the Americans with Disabilities Act (ADA) of 1990 are your primary lines of defense against job discrimination. The ADA protects people in private employment (businesses with more than fifteen employees), and the FRA offers the same protection for federal employees and people who work for companies that receive federal funding. In addition, there is a variety of state, county, and local laws that protect you against discrimination.

You probably don't think of yourself as disabled, and you shouldn't, but these laws scoop you up into their very capacious net that defines the disabled as anyone who has a physical or mental impairment that substantially limits one or more major life activities, has a history of such impairment, or is regarded as having such an impairment.

In general, these are the ways in which the laws protect you at work:

- An employer cannot exclude you from its group health insurance plan. If you work at a place where there are fewer than fifteen employees, you may be required to undergo a health screening examination. In that case, it is best to tell the truth about your diabetes and tell the examining physician how you control your glucose. It also wouldn't hurt to present a written statement from your physician telling your employer how healthy you are and how your diabetes will have no effect on your work performance.

- An employer cannot ask you for health or medical information until you are offered a job, and only if it asks all employees the same questions.
- Once you have started working, your employer may not ask medical questions unless it is related to your job performance.
- An employer is required to provide reasonable physical accommodations for people with disabilities such as wheelchair ramps and doorways that are wide enough to allow wheelchair access. For people with diabetes, these accommodations must include sufficient breaks to monitor blood glucose and take insulin injections and a private place in which to do it. You may also keep snacks and diabetes supplies near your work station.
- If you lie when asked a legally permissible question about your health, you lose the protection of the law.

To Tell or Not to Tell

It is entirely up to you whether you tell people at work that you have diabetes, but you should be aware of one thing: Many people cannot keep secrets, and personal revelations told in absolute confidence have a way of leaking out sooner rather than later. It's not that people are evil or disrespectful or intend to hurt you, it's that they're are all human, and gossip is what it is: a natural and pleasurable human activity. So if you don't want everyone at work to know about your diabetes, tell no one. An advantage of not telling is that if no one knows you have diabetes, then they can't discriminate against you for it.

However, people make friends at work, lunchtime conversation often turns to personal topics, relationships with co-workers are often close and even intimate, and you might naturally want to take people into your confidence about something that you have integrated completely into your life and no longer see as so different, odd, or weird. Beware that others, however, might not see it that way, and people may suddenly begin to treat you differently and discriminate against you in a personal way.

If you are a Type I diabetic, especially if you have had serious hypo- or hyperglycemia in the past, it is a good idea to take an officemate or someone who works near you into your confidence so that if you run into trouble at work, that person will know how to help you. Also, if you use your glucose monitor or take insulin, sooner or later someone is going to see you, either in the bathroom or in your office. Coming upon a co-worker sticking a needle into their arm is a shock, and insulin is the last thing people will think it is. It might be less stressful to prepare fellow employees than to be put into the humiliating position of having to prove to the bosses that you are not a drug addict.

Another reason to tell co-workers about your diabetes is that you can educate them about the disease, both for their own good and so that if they had a tendency to discriminate against you, they will be less likely once they know more about it. Then again, perhaps it won't make a difference one way or the other, and you may not consider it part of your responsibility to teach people about your disease and prepare others for the eventuality of also getting it.

One last thing: By telling co-workers and personal friends that you have diabetes, you find out who your friends really are. Those who curl their lip and walk away are obviously not in that category. It's up to you to decide whether it's better not to know.

Joyce thinks everyone should be completely open about having diabetes, and says it increases her self-esteem by not having to keep secrets about such an important thing. She also educates everyone she comes in close contact with about diabetes. Her partner, Hal, also has diabetes, but he doesn't tell anyone. They've both chosen different ways to approach their management of diabetes in their lives.

Fighting Discrimination

In general, most attorneys will tell you that there are three steps in fighting discrimination: education, negotiation, and litigation. It is not within the scope of this book to go into detail about how to fight discrimination (you need a lawyer or the federal Equal Employment Opportunities Commission for that; the American Diabetes Association Attorneys Network consists of about seventy attorneys who have expressed interest in helping people with diabetes who have been treated unfairly—contact your state or local chapter for a referral).

There are, however, things you should do. The first is to document everything. Put everything that happens to you in writing as soon as it happens. Note the date, the time, the people involved (including witnesses), and who said what to whom. You don't have to show these documents to anyone if the problem is resolved and nothing further happens, but don't throw them out. You never know what the future will bring. A good idea is to make two copies of each document. Keep one in a safe place at home and put the other in an envelope and mail it to yourself at home. When you receive it, don't open the envelope; the postmark will be proof that the incident happened when you said it did. If the incidents escalate, your stack of envelopes will make an impressive case on your behalf.

One of the first things you should do if you intend to sue your employer for discrimination is to document the fact that your diabetes is in good control. This documentation takes two forms: your own records and those of your physician. You should be keeping a written record of your blood glucose tests, which can be used as proof that not only are you in good control but you take care of yourself and follow the prescribed regimen. Then, you can ask your physician to support your claim that your diabetes does not make you a menace to anyone at work. Ask for a letter to that effect, perhaps including recent glycohemoglobin results.

Other steps to take when you have been discriminated against are to educate your employer and co-workers about diabetes so they can understand that they have no reason to think you are less capable than anyone else and thus are equally deserving of a raise or promotion—or of not being fired. If that doesn't work, you should point out that what they are attempting to do is illegal; show them in black and white the relevant passages from the ADA. Insist politely that you have certain rights that you will not permit them to abrogate. If that doesn't work, seek legal advice and sue them.

Military

The military is a tough nut to crack. Although the actual rules about diabetics in the military have eased somewhat, you still may not enlist if you already have the disease. If you contract it while you are on active duty, things are not as clear. Military physicians will make a decision about keeping you on or giving you a medical discharge. They base the decision on whether you have Type I or Type II, the kinds of medications you take, the amount of control you have over your blood glucose, and other factors.

When your diabetes is diagnosed, your case will be presented to a physical evaluation board, which declares you either fit or unfit for military duty. If you are fit, you may either return to your regular assignment or be transferred to another unit or type of work. If you are declared unfit, you are given a military discharge, which you can appeal.

Your chances of staying in the military are much better with Type II diabetes that is controlled without medication. If you need to take oral hypoglycemic agents, it's a bit more iffy. If you get Type I disease, you can pretty much count on having to pack your duffel bag.

If you are a Marine, you will be automatically given a medical discharge. This branch of the service requires every single serviceperson to be combat ready, regardless of one's current occupation in the Marines. Cooks, clerks, and generals all have to be ready to fight. The Air Force and Navy are fairly rigid about not allowing diabetics to remain on active duty, and the Army has the most inconsistently applied regulations.

Mike is in the Army and got a whopping case of Type I diabetes at age forty-three, an unusual thing to happen. At first the doctors didn't know what was wrong with him, since he wasn't overweight, he's physically fit, and he didn't fit the age profile. He had severe vision problems, and was essentially blind for about three weeks; he also had other symptoms of diabetes and a blood glucose of 540. That clinched it.

Mike was in the hospital for a while as his blood glucose was controlled and his insulin dosage regulated. Four months after diagnosis, he looks like the picture of health, his vision is fine, and his blood glucose is down to around 140. His case is before the medical review board right now. He's a recruiter, so he will never have to go to combat, but he doubts they'll let him stay in. He was really sick at the beginning, and he's on a complicated insulin-diet regulation program, so he thinks it's only a matter of time until he gets his medical discharge. He was almost ready to retire anyway. He has eighteen years in so the diabetes would push his discharge up two years; if he appeals, he could probably draw the process out for the two years—until he served his full twenty.

His pension would be 50 percent of his most recent base pay if he retired "naturally." With a medical discharge, he will receive only 30 to 40 percent of base pay. That's a significant difference, especially if he has a hard time finding work when he gets out of the Army. He has a wife and two children. Also, there is the stigma of being forced to leave the service involuntarily for something other than a combat-related illness.

Paying for Diabetes

Ways to Save Money

Much of your diabetes care is covered by health insurance, but some is not. However, even items that are covered (not including office visits to health professionals) require you to lay out the money first and then make a claim to be reimbursed. That can add up to a significant amount of out-of-pocket cash. Following are some ways you can reduce those expenses:

- Use syringes more than once. This is perfectly safe as long as you take precautions to maintain sterility, such as replacing the plastic cap that fits over the needle.
- Compare prices on brands of insulin. There may be a significant difference in price but no difference in quality.
- When taking oral hypoglycemic agents, ask your physician to prescribe a generic drug if there is one.
- Buy a glucose monitor, lancets, and test strips that offer a rebate. Shop around until you find one.
- Take care of all your equipment so that it will last as long as possible.
- When grocery shopping, stay away from prepared food and junk food. These are the most expensive items in the supermarket and are almost always lacking in the nutrition you need.

In Extreme Poverty

Diabetes is an expensive disease, even without complications, and if you are poor, you might be tempted to cut corners on blood glucose testing and medications. Don't. There are too many avenues of help for you to have to resort to jeopardizing your health.

There are a number of government, nonprofit, and voluntary clinics and other organizations, many of which are supported in whole or in part by pharmaceutical companies, that provide free or low-cost care for diabetics. It takes some time and effort to find them, but a few hours on the telephone should net you good results.

It's difficult, but have a frank discussion about money with your primary care physician. Some physicians will provide free samples of insulin or oral hypoglycemics. If your doctor doesn't volunteer, contact the pharmaceutical company yourself. They all have toll-free phone numbers for their customer relations department, and many will provide free drugs—at least for a while.

Next, try the federal government. If you are over sixty-five, you are on Medicare, which is now much more liberal about paying for diabetic supplies. If you are under sixty-five and have been disabled for at least twenty-four months by a complication of diabetes, you also may qualify for Medicare. If you have permanent kidney failure, you automatically qualify. Call and ask.

If you are a Medicare beneficiary and are having a hard time paying for your supplementary insurance (sometimes known as a Medigap policy), which pays for deductibles and copayments, the federal government can help. The new Qualified Medicare Beneficiary (QMB) program requires that state Medicaid pay Medicare costs for certain elderly and disabled people with low incomes and limited resources. If you qualify, Medicaid will pay all Medicare deductibles and copayments, as well as reimburse you for the monthly Medicare premium that Social Security deducts from your check each month. If this sounds confusing, it is a little. For more information, write to Consumer Information Center, Department 87, Pueblo CO 81009 and ask for a free copy of "Medicare: Savings for Qualified Beneficiaries." If you think you qualify for QMB, apply at your state or local Medicaid, welfare, social service, or public health office.

Call your state or county welfare office and find out if you are eligible for Medicaid and/or food stamps. In most states, if you earn more than $200 or $300 a month, you don't qualify, but it's worth a phone call. If you receive Aid to Families with Dependent Children (AFDC), Old Age Assistance (OAA), Aid to the Blind, Aid to the Permanently and Totally Disabled, or Supplemental Security Income (SSI), or if you are a nursing home resident, you will probably qualify for Medicaid.

Women, Infants, and Children (WIC) is a federal food grant program that provides food subsidies and nutrition counseling for pregnant women and high-risk children up to age five. Your local health department will have information on how to apply.

The Veterans Administration, which operates the largest health care system in the United States, serves veterans in two major categories: those who have service-related health problems and those who are indigent. You may qualify in the latter category. Call or visit your local VA office to find out.

Other sources of help include:

- *Food stamps.* Qualifications for food stamps are much less strict than for other aid programs. If you are poor and can prove it, you will probably get them. Call the local welfare office and find out how you need to document your indigence.
- *Nutrition advice.* Most local and county health departments have nutritionists on staff at least part time. The service is free.
- *Shelters and soup kitchens.* Many churches, synagogues, and other community groups provide free and nutritious meals. Don't let pride stand in your way of a good meal. When you are back on your financial feet, you can repay the debt by volunteering where you were fed.
- A variety of nonprofit organizations provide financial assistance to diabetics: the American Academy of Ophthalmology (800-222-EYES), the Benevolent and Protective Order of the Elks, Lions Club International, and others. The ADA Information and Action Line (800-DIABETES) can refer you to other sources of financial assistance.

11

Sexuality and Pregnancy

Sexual Function

It is commonly believed that diabetes interferes with sexual function, especially male potency. This is both true and false. Although most diabetics are able to have entirely satisfying sex lives, or at least as satisfying as before the disease was diagnosed, this is not to say that there will be no problems at all.

Some of the problems or issues are not related to the physical fact of diabetes. For example, if you are unduly depressed or anxious over having the disease, you may experience a diminished sex drive because of the depression or anxiety, not the diabetes. And if your diabetes is in poor control, and your blood glucose is too high a good deal of the time, you might suffer from feelings of hopelessness and helplessness, which decrease sex drive. And of course, hypoglycemia robs you of the energy you need for sex.

Women

Menstruation

Some diabetic women experience a rise in blood glucose two to four days before their menstrual period. This increase is due to elevated levels of estrogen and progesterone, probably because of an incompletely understood interaction between insulin and receptor sites on hormonal cells, which causes temporary additional insulin resistance. Some women, on the other hand, have a seemingly paradoxical effect: higher-than-normal estrogen levels improve insulin action and thus lower blood glucose. As soon as the flow begins, blood glucose evens out. However, Type I diabetics should tell their physicians about this, and you may need a slightly increased dose of insulin for these few days.

Other things you can do to keep you blood glucose normal during the premenstrual period include:

- Eat at regular intervals to prevent fluctuations in blood glucose.
- Avoid caffeine, chocolate, alcohol, and too much carbohydrate, which can affect blood glucose levels, as well as your emotions.
- Don't skip your exercise sessions and even add a little extra time and effort.

Yeast Infections

High blood glucose is one of the causes of vaginal yeast infections, which is how many women first discover that they have diabetes. In fact, if a woman over forty, who hasn't had a yeast infection since she was in her twenties, suddenly has recurring yeast infections, she should have her blood glucose checked professionally.

It is inadvisable to have sexual intercourse while you are being treated for a vaginal yeast infection. In the first place, you will feel so itchy from the infection and sticky from the topical creams and suppositories that you probably have no inclination to make love. But even if you did, you could transfer the infectious microbes to your sex partner.

Vaginal Dryness

Two phenomena are at work here. Diabetes itself sometimes causes vaginal dryness, and the age of onset of Type II diabetes often coincides with the approach or onset of menopause, which, because of decreasing amounts of estrogen, almost always results in the same problem.

Luckily, it is easy to remedy. Menopausal women who take hormone replacement therapy usually find that the medication resolves the problem. Women who do not choose hormone replacement can find relief from the discomfort of sexual intercourse with a variety of vaginal lubricants. Most people like Astroglide best, but you should buy several brands and experiment to see which is most pleasing to you and your sex partner. Do not use petroleum-based lubricants such as Vaseline or mineral oil or vegetable oils such as cooking oil, Crisco, or olive oil. None of these preparations are water soluble, and they will cling for days to your sensitive genital tissues. The best thing to do is go to a large well-stocked drugstore and spend some time reading the labels that specifically describe the product as a vaginal lubricant.

Menopause

Some women go through menopause with only a hot flash or two and no other symptoms, except the main one: no more menstrual periods. Others, however, are miserable for a year or two with frequent, searing hot flashes; irregular and often exceptionally heavy periods; depression; and all kinds of other unpleasant symptoms. If you are having serious menopausal problems, you should be under the care of a board-certified gynecologist who likes to care for older women (as opposed to those whose practice consists mainly of women in their childbearing years).

Even if you sail through the experience with hardly a backward glance, your hormones are undergoing the same changes as everyone else. Menopause is an entirely normal and natural phenomenon, but because your hormones have changed markedly, you are now at increased risk of cardiovascular disease and osteoporosis (a disease characterized by diminution in bone mass and density, which makes you more susceptible to fractures). This is also the age at which women start having a higher incidence of breast and reproductive organ cancer. As a diabetic, you have always been at increased risk of cardiovascular disease; now as a diabetic menopausal women, your risk zooms up.

For this and other reasons you may want to consider hormone replacement therapy (HRT): a combination of estrogen and progesterone that alleviates many of the symptoms of menopause and lowers the risk of cardiovascular disease and osteoporosis, although no one is certain how it does this. Although the decision to take HRT is entirely yours, you should discuss the pros and cons with your gynecologist because there are some downsides: HRT may cause irregular bleeding even after your natural periods have stopped, it may make you more insulin sensitive, and there has been an incredible amount of controversy in the medical and lay press about the relationship of HRT to the risk of breast and endometrial cancer. However, to date there has been no definitive proof one way or the other. Be sure to tell your gynecologist that you are diabetic.

Birth Control Pills

Birth control pills are hormones and come in three major types: monophasic, triphasic, and progesterone only. Monophasic pills contain a fixed amount of estrogen and progesterone and are taken every day of your menstrual cycle. Women whose blood glucose tends to fluctuate prior to menstruation may find that monophasic pills help even things out. Triphasic pills contain varying doses of estrogen and progesterone, which you take in sequence throughout your cycle. They may or may not affect your blood glucose. Experience will show you how you react to them. Progesterone-only contraceptives are available in pill, injectable, or implantable form.

Short-term studies have shown that all three types are safe for most diabetic women, but there is no research on the effects of oral contraceptives over the long haul. If you smoke, are over thirty-five, have a history of cardiovascular disease, have high blood pressure, and/or have peripheral neuropathy, you should not take oral contraceptives. If you decide to take oral contraceptives, be sure to tell your gynecologist that you are a diabetic.

Men

Impotence

Many men are more afraid of the possibility of impotence than they are of the side effects of diabetes. Impotence, defined as the inability to achieve or sustain an erection sufficient for sexual function, is a problem not just of diabetics but of all men. When a diabetic man suffers from impotence, the cause may or may not be related to the physicality of diabetes. In fact, the major cause of impotence in all men is psychological: tension, fear of the failure to perform sexually (often called performance anxiety), guilt, depression, grief—almost anything that preys on the mind.

In terms of physical causes of impotence, some are directly related to diabetes and some are not. Most diabetic impotence does not appear until a man has had the disease for many years, and then it is more likely to occur when the diabetes has not been well-controlled for a long time. No one knows exactly why impotence is associated with diabetes, but many physicians believe it is a form of neuropathy. Nerves that control erection are damaged as a result of chronically high levels of blood glucose. These nerves control tiny valves in blood vessels leading to and from the penis. When the valves open as a result of sexual stimulation, blood fills the vessels of the penis. They then close and trap the blood there, stiffening the penis. If the nerves that control these valves are damaged, erection is impossible. A major nondiabetic cause of impotence is the hardening or occluding of the vessels that supply blood to the penis, thus preventing a sufficient amount of blood flow to stiffen it.

Impotence is not a sudden occurrence. Most men notice that over time, their erection is not as hard as it used to be, or they cannot sustain it for long enough. Sexual desire is not diminished at all, which is what makes impotence so frustrating.

And because American men are so emotionally, socially, and culturally focused on sex and their ability to "perform," many of them are ashamed, embarrassed, and reluctant to talk about impotence, even with their sexual partners. There are, however, a number of ways that men can counteract or even solve the problem:

- Discuss the problem with your physician, because you need to find out the cause before you can correct it.
- Impotence may be a side effect of a medication, and discontinuing it or changing the brand or type of drug may solve the problem.
- Couples counseling or individual therapy can help you deal with the problem and, in the process, increase your ability to sustain an erection.
- A penile prosthesis, surgically inserted into the penis, can create the ability to have sexual intercourse. One type of prosthesis keeps the penis permanently erect, but it can be folded down during times other than sexual intercourse. The other type inflates when needed by means of a small pump located under a testicle. Both types of prosthesis have no effect on sperm production or the ejaculatory process; they have no reproductive repercussions.
- Nonsurgical mechanical devices exist as well. There is a vacuum device that fits over the penis and pulls blood into it. Another technique involves self-injection of a substance that constricts blood vessels, trapping blood in the penis for a temporary erection.

In early 1998, the FDA approved the first drug to treat impotency. Viagra (sildenafil) is taken about an hour before intercourse, acts on the physiological system in the penis, and causes an erection in a man who is sexually excited. It has no effect if the man is not aroused. The drug's manufacturer, Pfizer, claims that it will help 70 to 80 percent of impotent men. The most common side effect is headache; others include flushing, indigestion, and a stuffy nose.

Whether Viagra will work for diabetics depends on how badly the nerves of the penis have been damaged by elevated glucose over the years. The best course of action is to try it and see—but don't get your hopes up.

More important than treating impotence, which may be only temporary, is preventing it in the first place. The number of diabetics who eventually becomes impotent ranges from about 10 to 50 percent of men between age thirty and eighty. Because neuropathy is the main cause, maintaining tight blood glucose control can decrease the statistical risk of impotence.

Retrograde Ejaculation

Retrograde ejaculation, experienced by a few men with diabetes, is the backward flow of semen into the bladder at ejaculation. It is thought to be caused by nerve damage. Retrograde ejaculation may diminish reproductive capacity if none of the semen enters the vagina, and some men are psychologically disturbed by the lack of "evidence" that they have ejaculated.

Men and Women

There are a number of sexual and related problems that affect both men and women.

Urinary Tract Infections

Urinary tract infections (UTI) are much more common in people with elevated blood glucose. Various bacteria thrive in an atmosphere of increased sugar content, and the immune system is less able to combat the infection. UTIs tend to be uncomfortable and painful, and you should not have sex while you are being treated, even in the unlikely event that you want to. The infectious organisms are often contagious.

Genital Infections

Genital infections also are more common in diabetics. Men can get yeast infections too; they are usually related to poor blood glucose control and are as easily treated with topical creams and lotions as those of women.

Pregnancy

Although pregnant women with diabetes are considered high risk, their survival rate and that of their infants is the same as nondiabetic women. There are, however, things about which diabetic women need to be especially careful during pregnancy. You guessed it—the most important is keeping tight blood glucose control.

Deciding to become pregnant at any time is one of the most important decisions a woman can make. If she is diabetic, it is even more important because of two major factors: Your diabetes should be in excellent control before pregnancy begins, and you must make a commitment to keep it that way throughout the entire pregnancy. It can be difficult at times. There is no reason why you and your baby cannot come through the forty-week experience in fine health, but you should understand at the outset that there are risks you will take that nondiabetic women will not.

If you have complications of diabetes and are thinking of getting pregnant, you should first have a thorough medical and eye examination. Some complications worsen during pregnancy, although they usually even out after delivery. For instance, if you have diabetic retinopathy that has reached the stage where your ophthalmologist has noticed the formation of new blood vessels (neovascularization) in your eyes, you should think seriously about not becoming pregnant. You could go blind. Your kidneys are also especially vulnerable during pregnancy. If you find protein in your urine, postpone pregnancy until the problem is corrected because it could lead to serious hypertension.

Insulin requirements in nondiabetic women change during pregnancy because the placenta, which produces hormones of its own, makes insulin work less efficiently. In fact, by the last trimester, a pregnant woman requires (and her body manufactures) about twice as much insulin as needed in the nonpregnant state. Thus, if you took insulin before you became pregnant, you will likely need about twice as big a dose by the end. However, do not calculate your own insulin dosage. Your physician will decide how often and by how much to gradually increase your insulin dosage.

Think about what this hormone imbalance can do to a diabetic woman. A pregnant body that receives insufficient nutrients or other chemicals of any kind will use available stores of those nutrients or chemicals to nourish the fetus and maintain the pregnant woman's health. Therefore, if there is not enough insulin in the first place to help turn available sugar into energy, the body will use stored fat for energy and "give" stored protein to the fetus. When this happens, ketoacidosis can result.

In addition to more insulin, you will need to eat more calories and an increased amount of carbohydrates and protein, and you will need to keep a careful balance among food intake, physical activity, and medication (both insulin and oral hypoglycemics). The best way to do this is to put yourself in the care of a nutritionist for the duration of your pregnancy and the weeks immediately after the delivery. Most obstetricians who care for high-risk pregnancies can recommend a nutrition professional, and many have someone on staff.

Gestational Diabetes

In the event that a nondiabetic woman's pancreas cannot keep up with the extra insulin needed during pregnancy, she will develop gestational diabetes, a condition that almost always disappears after delivery. Gestational diabetes is more common in overweight women, those who have a family history of diabetes, and those who are over thirty when they become pregnant. Some cases of gestational diabetes are actually undiagnosed "regular" diabetes, which is then treated in the usual way.

Most gestational diabetes can be controlled by diet alone. Rarely is insulin needed, but if you do have to take it, it is discontinued after delivery. Gestational diabetes creates a higher risk for some of the "ordinary" complications of pregnancy such as toxemia.

Obstetrical Care

Some women, when they realize they are pregnant, wait a few months to begin prenatal obstetrical care. Diabetics should not do that. You must make an appointment with your obstetrician-gynecologist the minute you have confirmed your pregnancy (or as soon as you have missed your second menstrual period), and immediately tell the doctor that you are a diabetic. If the physician is not experienced in high-risk pregnancy, ask for a referral to someone who is. Don't be afraid of hurting your OBG's feelings. This is your health and that of your baby. You must do everything you can to take care of yourselves.

Women who live in a major metropolitan area may wish to be cared for during their pregnancy by a specialized team of experts, consisting of an endocrinologist, an ophthalmologist, a perinatologist (high-risk pregnancy specialist), a dietician, and a neonatologist (specialist in newborn infants). If you live far from such a center, you need to make certain that your primary care physician or endocrinologist is in frequent contact with your obstetrician about combining your two health issues: diabetes and pregnancy.

For the most part, your obstetrical care will be like that of nondiabetic women. There are, however, a few additions and differences: The first trimester, when you need weekly visits to the doctor, is the most critical to the health and development of the fetus; it is especially important to keep your diabetes in tight control during this time to prevent birth defects and intrauterine damage. You also need to reevaluate your diet with the guidance of a nutritionist who may suggest that you take vitamin and iron supplements. Your weight, blood pressure, and eyes should be checked frequently. If you suffer from morning sickness, your insulin dose may need to be adjusted to compensate for the food that you can't manage to keep down.

During the second trimester, you should keep up your weekly visits to the obstetrician. Often, diabetes stabilizes now, although you may have to increase your insulin. It becomes even more important during the middle trimester to monitor your blood pressure (it would be a good idea to buy a home blood pressure monitor and keep track of it yourself), fluid retention, kidney function, and hemoglobin (the component of red blood cells that carries oxygen to tissues).

Weekly visits to your physician are especially important during the third trimester. Even though your diabetes may be stable, especially if you've been conscientious about sticking to your food regimen, you may need more insulin. If your blood pressure were to rise suddenly, the third trimester is when it usually happens, and this is also the danger period for kidney problems and fluid retention.

In addition to fetal health checkups that all women receive (alfa-fetoprotein, ultrasound, nonstress test, oxytocin challenge test, and amniocentesis), there are special things that diabetic women need to monitor closely throughout pregnancy:

- *Urine.* Urine must be checked for ketones and the presence of bacteria, which could indicate a urinary tract infection.
- *Blood pressure.* This could prevent a condition called preeclampsia, common in diabetics during pregnancy and in the presence of gestational diabetes. Preeclampsia usually appears in the late stages of pregnancy and is characterized by high blood pressure and swelling of the feet and ankles. It can lead to a much more serious condition called eclampsia, which can cause seizures and harm to the fetus.
- *Blood glucose.* This should be done four times a day by self-monitoring and by regular professional blood testing.
- *Ketones.* You should monitor your ketone level every day by testing your urine.
- *Glucose control.* The most important thing for all diabetics, it is especially essential that pregnant women with diabetes maintain tight glucose control.

Food and Physical Activity

You will gain weight during your pregnancy. Everyone does. The weight is not just the fetus (although sometimes it feels like it); it is the additional blood your body produces to nourish the fetus, as well as additional tissue that support the fetus (breast enlargement, the placenta, amniotic fluid, and fat stores). If your weight was about right before you got pregnant, you will want to gain twenty-four to twenty-eight pounds. If you were too heavy, your physician may ask that you keep the weight gain down to fifteen to twenty-five pounds, and if you were underweight, you may need to gain twenty-eight to thirty-two pounds.

Try to gain your weight gradually, less in the first trimester and more in the second and third, and remember that although you may indeed be eating for two, the baby is nowhere near your size, so this does not mean double helpings of everything.

It's extremely important for you to keep up with a physical activity plan, although the kind of exercise may have to change for the duration. This is something you should discuss with your physician, although in general, you should stick to walking, swimming, and other exercises that don't require good balance (because your center of gravity has been thrown off) and that don't result in a lot of jiggling and bouncing around.

Delivery and Postpartum

Women with diabetes tend to have larger babies than nondiabetic women; a nine or ten pound baby is not unusual. In order to avoid the complications of delivering such a handful, or risking the necessity of a cesarean section, most diabetic women have their labor induced at about thirty-eight weeks—after undergoing an amniocentesis to make certain that the baby's lungs are mature.

On the morning of the scheduled delivery, you will check into the hospital and will receive only a small portion of your usual insulin dose, and during the time you are in labor, your blood glucose will be monitored frequently. Although labor is not considered an illness, it is extremely stressful and thus can cause strong fluctuations in glucose levels. Immediately after delivery, your insulin requirement will drop drastically, perhaps to even less than you needed before you became pregnant. But after a few days, things should even out, and you will probably be back to your prepregnant dose level.

Your baby may stay in the observation nursery of the hospital for a few days after you are discharged because sometimes babies of diabetic women have minor ailments not seen in babies of nondiabetic women. The pediatrician you have chosen will examine your new baby as soon as it is born, and if the hospital has a neonatologist on staff (most major medical centers with large labor and delivery units do), your baby will be the patient of that specialist during the hospitalization.

Breast feeding is perfectly fine for diabetic women, but you will need extra calories and additional carbohydrate—almost as much as when you were pregnant. Since milk production requires a great deal of nutritional energy, you need to discuss your new diet plan with a nutritionist. If you have managed to get this far without seeing one, now is the time when you really must. All hospitals have nutritionists on staff. Request a consultation.

12

Diabetes in Childhood

Characteristics of Childhood Diabetes

The causes of diabetes acquired in childhood (sometimes called juvenile diabetes) are approximately the same as they are in the disease acquired in adulthood. Boys and girls are equally likely to become diabetic.

The major difference between childhood and adult-onset diabetes is that the former is insulin dependent: Type I. Symptoms of childhood diabetes usually develop rapidly, whereas adults notice the problem more gradually. Also, the symptoms tend to be more severe: voracious thirst with frequent urination; a hugely increased appetite with concomitant weight loss; episodes of bed wetting; and blurry vision due to rapid change in the shape of the eyeball. In short, a normally active and healthy child suddenly becomes weak, listless, and irritable. A child's schoolwork may deteriorate, and there may be complaints of leg and/or abdominal pains.

The good news is that the diagnosis is easy to make—one blood test tells the story, and treatment can begin immediately. Your pediatrician will make the initial diagnosis, but it is important that you ask for a referral to a physician who specializes in childhood diabetes. Your pediatrician will, however, continue to care for your child's general health. But pediatricians are generalists and you need a specialist. Your child with diabetes also will require the services of other health care providers: a nutritionist, an ophthalmologist, a diabetes educator, and possibly a social worker or psychologist.

The stages of childhood diabetes are similar to the stages of Type I diabetes in adults:

- *Newly diagnosed.* The diabetes can probably be controlled with small doses of intermediate-acting insulin.
- *Remission.* There appears to be improvement in the disease, and only very small doses of insulin are required. Remission often ends with an acute infection, the onset of puberty, or other stressful event.
- *Intensification.* The diabetes appears to be getting worse (but is not) and is more difficult to control. Blood glucose must be monitored carefully and insulin dosage adjusted frequently.
- *Total diabetes.* Beta cells are completely destroyed, and your child is completely dependent on insulin.

Treatment of childhood diabetes is essentially the same as it is in adults: tight blood glucose control, relief of symptoms, and prevention of complications. However, there are unique emotional, practical, and social issues inherent in childhood diabetes. I will discuss them throughout this chapter.

Emergencies and Complications

Serious complications of diabetes in children are the same as they are in adults, but they usually don't show up until adulthood or adolescence. And as with adults, the tighter the blood glucose control, the less risk there is of serious complications.

There is no medical evidence to show that diabetic children fall ill or have more accidents than nondiabetic ones. They are no more likely to be hospitalized than anyone else. But kids are kids, and they all get sick and have accidents.

During nondiabetic illnesses and accidents, your first responsibility is to help the child recover from the illness because the longer the illness lasts, the more difficult it is to control blood glucose. But at the same time, during the illness you will have to help maintain as tight glucose control as you can. This is sometimes not so easy. Following are a few things that might help:

- If your child's appetite is so poor that food intake barely covers the insulin dose, give foods that are well tolerated and high in easily digested sugars: gelatin desserts, fruit and fruit juice, regular soda, crackers, tea with sugar, Gatorade and other sports drinks, ice cream, fruit yogurt, etc. Make certain your child drinks plenty of fluids: at least a half cup every hour.

- Offer food often. It is better to eat a little at a time than to force a whole meal down a sick child and have it come right back up.
- If your child will not or cannot eat at all, consider this an emergency and call the doctor. If the child is vomiting and/or tests positive for ketones, go to the emergency room without delay.
- Never stop giving insulin, even if the child is vomiting.

Food

As with adults, a diabetic child's nutritional needs are basically the same as those of children who do not have diabetes. If this sounds too easy to be true, it is—and it isn't. Meal planning, which a nutritionist can help you with, should not have to change much as long as your family was eating correctly in the first place. If not, then all of you will benefit from paying greater attention to the nutritional value of what you eat.

Children's meal plans should be reviewed about once a year because their needs change as they grow. In general, a child of average weight needs about one thousand calories a day at age one, with an additional one hundred calories a day added each year until the onset of puberty—at which time their caloric needs are the same as an adult.

There are really only two potential glitches in keeping your child on track in terms of food. The first is the need to coordinate food with insulin injections, and the second is the appalling eating habits of children when they are out of their parents' sight.

Regarding the first, insulin injections should be matched to eating times using the same principles as adults. To minimize a precipitous drop in blood glucose, the child should have snacks between meals and at bedtime. Meals and snacks should be eaten at about the same time every day—just as adults should. This is not usually a problem during the week when home and school meals are fairly tightly scheduled.

School lunches may not be the tastiest in the world, but they are nutritionally sound, and you can request a confidential conference with the school nutritionist who can then make certain that your child eats properly without creating special attention. If you pack a lunch, you have even more control. Snacks might be a little more problematic because most schools do not permit children to eat in the classroom or at other than designated lunchtime. In this case, you will need to go to school and arrange with the administration to obtain permission for your child to eat a snack when necessary.

Which brings you to the second problem: Kids often don't eat what their mothers pack in their lunch pails. They trade with other children, they throw it in the garbage and eat junk food, and for various reasons they sometimes skip lunch.

Eating is one of the many things that is subject to peer pressure during childhood. Children need to feel as though they are fully integrated members of their peer group, and being different in any way (too fat, too thin, wearing eyeglasses, having any physical deformity, even having the "wrong" haircut) is anathema to a child. If a child sees the diabetic food plan as in any way weird, it might be thrown out—to prove that the child is no different from anyone else.

It is also in the nature of children to test limits: to perform daredevil feats the minute they are out of their parents' sight, to get their ears pierced, to dye their hair orange, to stay out later than they are allowed. In fact, they will do almost anything they can get away with. This is a normal part of growing up: reaching for independence and testing the waters of the larger world. They will do it with their diabetic food plan, too. To see how far they can push their blood glucose levels to dangerous limits, they may balk at taking insulin (and when they are old enough to give themselves injections, they may skip doses), and they may stuff themselves with heavily sugared foods—just to see what will happen. They'll get into trouble as a result, which is why it is so important that you and they learn what to do in case of emergency.

Now that I have thoroughly terrified you about your child and food, I should say that things are not so bad. First, a food plan is only a guide—suggestions, within limits, of what your child should and should not eat. The more relaxed you are about that guide, the more relaxed your child will feel and the less hemmed in by a rigid food regimen. And the less rigid, the less the likelihood of rebellion against the whole thing—with resultant diabetic trouble. The ADA Guidelines lists the foods in categories from which you can make exchanges to create flexibility and variety (see appendix).

Naturally, your child will be angry about having diabetes, perhaps even at you. Angry children are unhappy children, so it is better to relax the food rules as much as possible than to create even more anger at having to stick to a diet.

Exercise

Exercise works the same in childhood diabetes as it does in the adult disease: It lowers blood glucose. Most children are very physically active, but if yours prefers to sit at home and read or watch television, you will have to devise a regular exercise program. Not calisthenics or enforced walking (that would probably not fit in with what a child thinks is appropriate), but group activities and sports. Following are some ideas about how you can increase children's physical activity:

- Teach them to ride a bicycle.
- Encourage participation in neighborhood after-school games.
- Sign them up for Little League or other organized community activity.
- Speak with the physical education teacher about ways to increase activity.

Diabetic children can participate in even the most strenuous sports and games as long as they eat extra carbohydrates before and after heavy exercise. If your child makes the team, which travels to other schools for games, don't discourage it. Rather, be proud of the achievement and again, use this as a learning experience on the road to independence. Make certain the child has enough food to cover all meals and snacks (pack a little extra just in case), write out a plan for how much carbohydrates to eat before and after the games, and make certain the coach and at least one other adult knows about the diabetes. Also, have your child pick a friend, someone who will be responsible enough to notify an adult, who can act as a "buddy" in case of hypoglycemia.

The only kind of exercise a diabetic child should avoid are those which are done totally alone: swimming or skiing alone, scuba diving, skydiving, etc.

Away from Home

School

Diabetic school children have to deal with a good deal of emotional stress, especially when they are first diagnosed. On one hand, they hate to appear different from their mates. On the other, they must keep their diabetes in control so they don't suffer physical consequences and end up in the nurse's office, or worse, have to be picked up by an ambulance in the school yard.

Luckily, after the first few weeks, this does not present a serious problem because glucose testing and insulin injections can be done at home at breakfast, supper, and bedtime. Children should carry a SBGM monitor with them to school, which can be easily hidden in their backpacks or even stuffed in a pocket. That's if they feel the need to hide it.

Laura is a nurse in a middle school (sixth, seventh, and eighth grades) and in her many years of knowing diabetic youngsters, she has never seen teasing or discrimination from diabetics' classmates. "The other kids are curious about the disease and the glucose monitor, but it's not malicious curiosity. They just want to know. Once they understand what's going on, they drop it. It's no more out of the ordinary than wearing glasses or wearing a leg brace." Laura said that the kids at her school seem to be nicer to each other than when she was young—and a lot nicer to each other than their parents are.

An important parental task is dealing with school administration and teachers. It is best to have these conferences in person after school so your child's friends don't see you there. The principal and other administrators, as well as all of your child's teachers and athletic coaches, must be told that your child has diabetes, and these adults need to understand what the disease is, what emergencies can arise, and what actions to take if they do.

Matthew and his mother never had problems with school authorities. Matthew's mother went to school as soon as he got out of the hospital after he was diagnosed (at age ten) and told everyone what she expected of them. She also told them that they were to let her know if Matthew appeared sick or not quite right in any way. She is a friendly no-nonsense woman with the demeanor of someone who expects to have reasonable requests granted. And so she did. Once she got a call from the physical education teacher. He said that Matthew didn't seem to have the sparkle that he usually did, so she went out and bought small cans of orange juice and took them to the school. She had the coach keep them in his locker and instructed him to let Matthew have a drink whenever he needed it.

Her advice to parents is to make sure that they don't stop their lives just because their children have diabetes. She explains that diabetes is not a good thing to have but it's not the worst thing in the world either. Matthew seems to feel the same way. He says having diabetes is a nuisance sometimes, since you have to remember to take all your diabetes stuff with you when you go over to someone's house or out of town with the team, and you can't eat some things, but he doesn't let it bother him all that much.

He has forgotten to take his insulin injections a few times, and he doesn't test his blood glucose as often as he probably should, but he keeps his diabetes in good control and he says he feels great. He looks terrific—tall, muscular, and blond.

Matthew, his three siblings, and his parents own and operate a 150-acre farm. They have 150 head of cattle, a herd of geese, three dogs, and about a half dozen cats. He says being responsible for the animals has taught him how to be responsible for himself. And he thinks that living outside has helped his diabetes, since working on the farm is good exercise. He explains that it's not like jogging once a day and then sacking out for the rest of the time. He gets constant activity.

He doesn't think of diabetes in terms of having a disease. He feels it's more like having to use crutches: it's something you have, but you learn to accept it and live with it.

In addition to making known what you want from school authorities, you should extract a promise from them that they will keep your child's diabetes confidential. For safety's sake, you must inform the adults who are responsible for them during the day, but it would be entirely unacceptable for these people to "tattle on" your child and make him the object of derision in front of his friends and schoolmates. Your child is the only one who is entitled to decide who to tell.

Of course, most children cannot keep a secret, so when you discuss this issue with your child, be certain you say that two seconds after a friend is told, the entire school may know. Your child probably won't believe you, but at least you have given the warning.

On the other hand, you assuredly don't want your child treated like an invalid or kept out of regular school activities. That is discrimination and federal laws exist to remedy it: Section 504 of the Rehabilitation Act of 1973, which protects people with disabilities against discrimination in any federally funded program, including public schools; and the Education for All Handicapped Children Act of 1975, which was amended in 1990 and is now called the Individuals with Disability Education Act. Diabetic children are specifically mentioned in the latter law because diabetes is considered a chronic health condition.

According to the law, all public schools must accommodate the needs of diabetic children, and a specialized individualized education plan must be developed for each handicapped child. You should discuss the plan with school administrators and teachers so that it will be truly individualized for your child. Elements of the plan include: eating wherever and whenever it is necessary; trips to the bathroom or water fountain during class; participation in field trips and extracurricular activities; increased days of absence; and assistance with blood glucose monitoring or insulin injections if the child needs it.

If your child is being discriminated against in any of these ways, fight it. Begin in a low-key manner by going to school to find out if the administration knows what is happening; often the principal has little idea of what goes on in classrooms. If the administration does know but doesn't care, step up your level of insistence on your child's rights. See chapter 10 for ways to handle discrimination, and be sure the lawyer you hire is experienced.

If you think discrimination in school is a thing of the past, think again. A survey of parents with diabetic children in the September 1995 issue of *Diabetes Forecast* revealed that teachers and school administrators have a long way to go in learning about diabetes—and in treating children with care and respect. That article provided the following information:

- 24 percent said that the school lunch program does not meet diabetic meal plan requirements
- 22 percent said that the school is inflexible about lunchtime
- 17 percent said their children don't have enough time to eat
- 24 percent said that their children are required to take exams when they are under the influence of hypo- or hyperglycemia

- 23 percent reported times when a hypoglycemic child was left alone
- 18 percent said that glucagon is not allowed in school
- 15 percent said that hypo- or hyperglycemia is not permitted to be treated in the classroom
- 13 percent of children are not allowed to eat snacks in the classroom
- 14 percent of children are not allowed to go to the bathroom or get a drink of water when they need to

Camp

If you are thinking of sending your child to overnight camp, you have two choices: regular camp or a camp for diabetic children. There are advantages and disadvantages of each.

A special camp for diabetic children can teach children more about diabetes; they are never seen as odd or different because everyone else is in the same boat (most of the counselors are also diabetic), and the environment is as safe as possible because everyone there is on the alert for diabetic emergencies. Children are away from their parents and can thus develop confidence in controlling their diabetes on their own without being isolated from helpful support. The summer can be a kind of support group. For a list of camps and Outward Bound programs for diabetic children, ask for a camp directory from the American Diabetes Association.

Regular camp is much like school, in that your child will probably be one of only a few diabetics—or the only one. An advantage of regular camp is that it mimics real life where diabetics are in the minority. In that sense, camp is good training for adult life, but it also can be lonely and isolating because at camp, everyone will know about the diabetes and everyone will witness glucose testing and insulin injections. There is no privacy at overnight camp.

On the other hand, your child might be a star because of the "oddity" of diabetes. Children like excitement, "coolness," and "weirdness," all of which they can attribute to a child with diabetes. It all depends your child's age, maturity, and desires.

Emotional Factors

Childhood diabetes has been described as feeling like a bomb that goes off in a family. In some respects this is an apt description because lives are forever altered and no one escapes the fallout. But unless the family was falling apart to begin with, the bomb analogy is too strong. Walls don't cave in, the foundation remains intact, and for the most part, relationships don't change.

There's no denying, however, that a big scary thing has happened and most families need to regroup and reassess the way they function in order to cope. Some families are so stressed out by childhood diabetes that eventually they need family therapy, but most manage. Many parents say that joining a support group provided the best help they found. Not only were they able to learn about diabetes in both formal and informal ways, but they slowly came to the point where they were able to help others. "It felt wonderful to be an 'old-timer,'" said one father as he looked back on a year of spending every other Wednesday evening in the basement of a Presbyterian church. "Those people helped Marge and me a lot—they'll never know how much. And now it feels good to be able to share what we know with people whose children have just been diagnosed."

Children with diabetes and their parents and siblings may be hurt, angry, guilty, and afraid. They wouldn't be human if they weren't. But feelings like these need to be expressed, and the family is the appropriate place to do it. Therefore, it is crucial that the child sit down with parents and siblings, with individual family members alone and in a family group, to talk about feelings in a reasonably calm and measured manner.

Feelings, no matter how negative, must be brought out into the open, or they will fester inside and "leak out" in inappropriate ways at inappropriate times. It is your responsibility to elicit feelings from your child, not the other way around. Saying, "It must feel like a drag sometimes not to be able to eat everything the other kids do," or "I bet sometimes you wish you could chuck the insulin out the window," will prompt a discussion, even perhaps a short burst of temper. This is far better than leaving the child to sulk and think that no one understands.

From the very beginning, children with diabetes need to be guided toward self-management, but they cannot be pushed. Guidance should be positive: "What do you think Johnny's mother will have for supper tomorrow night?" rather than, "Remember, you can't have dessert when you're at Johnny's tomorrow;" or "Don't forget to put your snacks in your gym bag for the game," rather than, "If you forget to eat your extra carbohydrate before the game you'll fall on your face on the field, and won't you be embarrassed."

Very young children can be encouraged to express their feelings as game-playing or play-acting. They can give pretend shots to their teddy bears and talk to their dolls about blood glucose testing. Insulin syringes without needles can be used as playthings so the child will get used to handling them. In addition to eliciting feelings, these activities can develop the habit of taking an active role in diabetes management.

On the other hand, you don't want your child to become diabetes obsessed. One can carry blood glucose testing, timing of meals, and interest in diabetes paraphernalia too far. I have met many diabetics whose entire lives revolved around their disease. It was almost all they talked about, and this is not the attitude you want to instill in your children.

If you don't want your child to grow up this way, try to keep a sense of balance and humor about having diabetes. Yes, diabetic children have to learn how to take care of themselves, but they also have to grow into fully developed human beings who must make their way in the big bad world—where diabetes usually is not a topic for discussion. Diabetes control is a learned skill, like balancing a checkbook, operating a computer, and finding and keeping a job. But it should not be the dominant part of one's life. You as the parent bear the bulk of the responsibility to help your child learn these things.

Childhood Diabetes by Age Group

Infants and Toddlers

Although it is not common, childhood diabetes is increasingly seen in children under age five. They require very small amounts of insulin, which of course parents must inject, usually in a diluted solution of U-100 regular insulin. A diabetes educator will show you how to prepare it.

Because the disease is so unusual in young children, it may not be diagnosed until your child is very ill with dehydration and fever. Hospitalization for a few days might be necessary while the disease is stabilized.

After discharge, the child may be thin and cranky and have a poor appetite. Insulin injections, blood tests, and other procedures will increase the moodiness. But once the disease is stabilized, and this happens very quickly, full appetite and sunny disposition return. Caring for an infant or toddler with diabetes is not as difficult as you might imagine.

A baby or toddler's urine is easy to test for glucose by squeezing a few drops from a diaper onto a test strip. (It is best not to test a baby's blood glucose except when absolutely necessary to avoid the repeated trauma of skin pricks.) Urine testing for glucose is not as accurate as blood testing, but it can give you a warning sign that all is not well. Often, the first sign of illness in an infant or toddler is elevated glucose. You should probably test your baby's urine several times a day for glucose (use a disposable diaper to avoid confounding the results with detergents).

When your child is first diagnosed, the doctor will suggest that you test for ketones several times a day; when the baby's diabetes is stabilized, once a week is usually often enough. If you need to test an infant or toddler's blood, use an earlobe rather than a finger. It is less traumatic and easier to get a drop of blood. Make sure the lobe is warm. Right after a hat is removed is a good time, or you might want to make a game of it by placing your hand over the child's ears and cooing or doing something else silly and fun.

One thing you should be aware of: An infant or toddler is too young to recognize the warning signs of hyper- or hypoglycemia, so you need to commit the symptoms to memory and be especially watchful. Toddlers are at a stage where they try to exert their independence, and if they don't feel like eating, they'll do just about anything to avoid it, including spitting out whatever you put in their mouths. Depending on their activity level, this might pose a problem. A flexible eating schedule can avoid food battles and reduces the risk of hypoglycemia. In addition, parents need to learn the difference between age-appropriate contrariness and other normal toddler behavior, and insulin reactions.

If a young child has an insulin reaction and is unconscious or won't take sugar by mouth, inject 1/2 cc of glucagon into the buttocks until the child is alert enough to take food by mouth. If there is no response in fifteen minutes, give another 1/2 cc and call the doctor.

Regarding babysitters, if you go out for an evening, it's probably unlikely that you will have to entrust a sitter with either blood glucose testing or insulin injections. But all babysitters should know the warning signs of hyper- and hypoglycemia and what actions to take, as well as what to do in the event of a diabetic emergency.

When hiring a babysitter, look for a responsible adult, not the thirteen-year-old down the street—unless it's a mature teenager with diabetes. They know what to look for and will be especially observant. It will give a teenager a boost in pride to think that parents of a diabetic baby have enough faith in their maturity to take responsibility for their child.

You should list all the signs and the actions to take for each and place it in a prominent place: near phones in the kitchen and family room or on the refrigerator—wherever your family's message center is located. The telephone number of your child's physician should be at the top of the list. In addition, you need to make certain that the babysitter knows where you will be at all times. Some parents carry a beeper, but this may be excessive.

It's a good idea for the babysitter to know how to give an insulin injection (you may time your evening out for between injections, but things happen and you might not be able to get home in time). Leave snacks for the baby with clearly written instructions of when and how they are to be given to the child. One way to solve the problem of having to teach a stranger all these things is to arrange a babysitting pool with other parents of diabetic children.

If both parents work outside the home, day care can be a problem. Most day care centers are not equipped to handle diabetic children; in fact, most won't take a child with any type of illness. So your options are limited. The best solution is again a pool of parents, but if you live in a small town, there probably won't be enough people.

Following are a few general pieces of information that might prove useful when caring for a little one with diabetes:

- When your baby cries or seems unusually fretful, the only way to know the difference between hypoglycemia and something else is to test blood glucose. If you are in a place where you absolutely cannot monitor blood glucose (or if you have forgotten to bring the monitor with you), give the baby some juice or a sugary snack. It is better to err on the side of too high than too low blood glucose.

- The best insulin syringes for babies are low-dose disposables that measure only up to fifty units and use U-100 insulin.
- Rotate injection sites to avoid lumps and depressions under the skin. Keep insulin at room temperature to make injections more comfortable.
- Both parents (and siblings if they are old enough) should give insulin injections so the baby does not see only one person as diabetes caretaker.
- Infants and toddlers must eat relatively soon after an injection, even if they don't want to. Think about devising creative ways to get your child to eat. Small snacks are probably better than large, regular meals so keep hard boiled eggs, fruit, and crackers on hand.
- If babies vomit after injections, they must eat something with enough carbohydrates to prevent an insulin reaction that won't upset their stomach. Regular soda or Popsicles are good.
- Read the label of commercial baby foods; most have added sugar. Many parents prefer to make their own baby food in a blender or food processor. Try freezing it in an ice cube tray that is separated into individual cubes; you can warm up the amount you need in the microwave and save the rest of the tray for another time.
- When you travel with your child, even if it's only a quick run to the supermarket, always have snacks, a bottle of insulin, and injection equipment with you.

Middle Childhood

Most youngsters in this age group can master at least part of their own diabetes management. Seven- or eight-year-olds can use a blood glucose monitor, and by age eight or so can be taught to give their own insulin injections. But don't rush children into taking too much responsibility too soon; let them be children while they are children.

Children ages six to twelve start to develop emotional independence, their motor skills are good, they can read and do easy math, and they are rapidly learning how to think analytically and reason. Therefore, they can choose and prepare their own snacks, with supervision, and make appropriate choices about what they eat—again, with guidance.

At this age, there can be incentives in learning to be responsible for one's own diabetes care: sleepovers at friends' homes, overnight camp, school trips, and the like. A child who is dependent on parents for all aspects of diabetes care can't participate fully in childhood activities.

One mother said that she used the same techniques to teach her eleven-year-old to take his own insulin that she used on her three-and-a-half-year-old to help him get toilet trained. "I reminded Jamie that if he was still in diapers and didn't tell me when he had to go, he wouldn't be allowed in the community swimming pool that summer. That snapped him out of his laziness about using the toilet! And I simply informed Sam that if he wanted to go on the weekend camping trip with his Boy Scout troop, he'd have to give himself the shots. Up until then, he could do everything but stick the needle in, but a week before the scouts were ready to hit the road, he screwed up his courage and did it. He really wanted to go on that trip."

Even when children are taking most of the responsibility for their own care and seem to be doing well with their food plan, parents still need to supervise. You don't have to hang over your child and demonstrate all the anxiety you're really feeling, but you do have to make certain that they're getting it right. Children of that age may not want to eat snacks that require special preparation and thus draw attention to themselves, so you need to pack things in their school bags that can be consumed inconspicuously in the classroom: granola bars, peanut butter and cheese crackers, animal crackers, and such.

You should not expect difficulty with your child's growth patterns as long as the insulin dose is correct and metabolism is normal. If you do notice growth retardation, tell the doctor; there are reasons other than diabetes for this problem.

Adolescence

This is the time when children will begin to accept full responsibility for managing their diabetes. A young person with a driver's license, a pack of college applications in a folder, and a tuxedo or prom dress should be responsible for all aspects of diabetes care—still with occasional parental supervision and the knowledge that if trouble crops up, you will be there to help.

Adolescence is a time of testing one's limits: outright rebellion, stubbornness, rapid vacillation between maturity and childishness, hand-wringing anxiety and adult composure, tears and laughter. This is completely normal, but the teenage years can and will have an effect on diabetes, which may be somewhat more difficult to control for a number of reasons:

- Teenagers' hormones undergo rapid and drastic changes.
- They often rebel against the values they grew up with, which might include what their parents have taught them about diabetes care.
- They tend to test the limits of what is socially appropriate and acceptable, and they often stretch common sense to its outermost boundary.
- Adolescents hate being different from their friends and associates and therefore might reject any part of diabetes care that they see as "different," which is almost all of it.
- Adolescents are champion sleepers and often do not get out of bed until noon or later on weekends. Diabetics can't be allowed to do this because they cannot miss meals, snacks, and insulin injections. But you can compromise with them: letting them sleep an hour later than usual, making sure they take their insulin and eat breakfast, and then sending them back to their room to sleep or laze about until the rest of their pals are awake.

Some of this behavior is acceptable and temporary and can probably be moderated with parent-child conversations or family conferences, but if you notice your teenager doing things that are clearly dangerous or self-destructive, you must get help: psychological counseling or family therapy.

If your adolescent girl's diabetes is in poor control, menarche (onset of menstruation) may be delayed for a while. Although this may be anxiety-producing for her, if her thyroid gland and other hormones are functioning normally, she will begin to menstruate as soon as her disease is in better control. Moreover, delayed menarche may act as a spur for her to take better care of herself.

This is also the time when children can start going to the doctor alone; therefore, their relationship with their parents will change. They will discuss things that you may never know about (a physician told something in confidence may not reveal it), and your teenager may make decisions with the physician that you had no part in. This will be hard for you to accept but probably no more difficult than watching your kids go out on dates.

They are separate people. They always have been, of course, but now they are becoming capable of living separate from you. They are now responsible for their own diabetes management.

Many adolescent activities revolve around food, so teenage diabetics need flexible meal plans that allow them to eat the way their peers do. There are many popular foods that can be fitted into diabetic meal plans: pizza, small hamburgers, diet soda, even french fries.

Teenagers also are old enough to plan their day and think about how much insulin they will need to cover their activities during the day. At first, you can go over their plans the night before, but by the time they are juniors and seniors in high school, they should be able to figure things out themselves. After all, in only a year or two, they'll probably be on their own in a college dorm or apartment.

Children, Adolescents, and the DCCT

Treating children and adolescents with diabetes used to focus on keeping blood glucose in reasonably good control while steering them through their various hormonal and psychosocial changes and illnesses. Glucose control was important but secondary.

With the conclusive results of the Diabetes Control and Complications Trial, that has changed. It is now known that glucose control is the most important factor in preventing long-term complications of diabetes, and this applies to adolescents as well as adults. Of the trial participants, 14 percent (195) were age thirteen to seventeen, all of whom were insulin dependent. When the study began, it was assumed that these kids would respond differently because they were experiencing a sharp rise in growth hormone and other growth factors that are chemically similar to insulin. It was therefore gratifying to find that the adolescents' response to intensive versus conventional diabetes therapy was similar in adolescents and adults, especially in terms of risk of microvascular changes that affect eyes and kidneys.

Adolescents in the trial also had the same adverse effects of intensive therapy as did adults: risk of weight gain and severe hypoglycemia. In fact, the rate of hypoglycemia in adolescent participants was higher than that of adults, but there were no long-term negative consequences of hypoglycemic episodes. The investigators believe that this higher risk of hypoglycemia is probably due, at least in part, to adolescents' greater irregularities in exercise and food intake, but the larger insulin doses required by younger people also may have played a role.

The results of the DCCT underscore the importance of spreading insulin doses throughout the day for strict glucose control. Reasonably good control can be achieved by some teenagers with two injections a day, but control is better and safer with three or more injections. Of course, the practical problem is to get kids to try a multiple-dose program. An insulin pump would be an ideal way to deliver insulin, but most teenagers find it too inconvenient and embarrassing.

The DCCT did not include children younger than thirteen years old, but extrapolating from the data and from what is known about younger children's physiology and biochemistry, most physicians believe that intensive therapy is less beneficial than conventional therapy for children younger than thirteen, especially infants and toddlers. They appear to be relatively well protected against eye and kidney changes with conventional therapy, and severe hypoglycemia is especially dangerous for brain development in younger children. Little kids, because their food intake and activity levels are so unpredictable, are particularly prone to severe hypoglycemia.

The more often blood glucose is monitored, and the more closely insulin dosage is tailored to the results, the less the risk of hypoglycemia and the better the glucose control.

13

Parenting a Child with Diabetes

Parental Roles and Responsibilities

You were probably floored when you found out that your child has diabetes. When you recovered from the shock, you may have experienced plenty of other emotions: anger, guilt, fear, and depression. These kinds of reactions are entirely normal. But as you work through your feelings (with or without professional psychological help), there are practical things you need to learn and do in order to take care of your child—and to help your son or daughter cope with the shock of having a serious illness at so young an age.

You may be feeling overwhelmed by what seems to be an enormity of details, and it will take a while to learn the intricacies of diabetes management and treatment and to teach them to your child. You don't have to do everything right away, but there are a few basic skills you need to get down pat as soon as you can:

- Monitoring blood glucose levels
- Giving insulin injections
- Recognizing and responding to hypo- and hyperglycemia
- Creating a menu and preparing your child's food based on the plan provided by a nutritionist

- Supervising physical exercise and moderating it based on insulin and food intake
- Knowing what to do when your child gets sick

Telling Your Child about Diabetes

Your child needs to be told about the diabetes as soon as you find out. It is natural to want to protect children from the unpleasant aspects of life, and diabetes is certainly something you would have preferred didn't happen. But it did happen and you will need to face it and live with it—as a family.

You really don't have a choice about whether to tell your child or when to do so. Insulin treatment has to begin right away; there's no getting around that. Also, your child knows there is something wrong and is probably as scared as you are, so the sooner you provide reassurance that this illness is something that can be treated and controlled, the sooner you can alleviate the fear. This is not to say that your child won't have all kinds of emotional reactions to having diabetes, but fear of the unknown will not be one of them, at least not as far as knowing what's wrong (fear of the future is always an issue with diabetics of any age).

Parents know their children best, and they can make the best guess about how their children will react, but most find that the best way to break the news is as gently and directly as possible. Age and emotional maturity make a big difference in how and what you tell your child about diabetes, but whatever amount of information you impart, make certain that it is accurate. Naturally, you will have to repeat things over and over again because children, like adults, don't generally remember details of a stressful event. And being told you have a serious illness is extremely stressful no matter how old you are.

How Your Reactions Affect Your Child

The way you react to and handle problems of daily life has a profound effect on the way your children perceive those problems and the way they eventually learn to cope with and solve problems as adults. Therefore, if you as a parent lose your cool and treat childhood diabetes as if it were a major disaster with guaranteed dire consequences, your child is going to fall into a panic and behave in ways that are counterproductive to treatment.

If, on the other hand, you treat the diabetes as if it were nothing more than a bad cold, and if you don't educate yourselves, your child will probably not learn how to manage the diabetes in a responsible and sensible manner. If you deny the significance and danger of diabetes, you will induce the same denial in your child, who will not learn good blood glucose control.

Children with diabetes may worry more than other children, and no wonder. They are under both physical and psychological threat, they have important responsibilities that the majority of their peers do not, and they learn that if they don't take care of themselves, the consequences can be dire. Therefore, you need to be sympathetic without becoming overprotective. Overprotective parents will create a fearful and overly dependent child.

If blame is tossed around the household like a malevolent football, everyone suffers. Even if you believe the diabetes comes from your spouse's side of the family, don't say it. There's enough guilt there already. And whatever you do, don't blame your child ("I told you not to eat so many candy bars"). There is absolutely nothing anyone could have done to prevent this. Therefore, casting blame is useless, pointless, and cruel.

The best approach goes something like this: "Diabetes is serious, but we can handle it, just as we've handled other problems in the past. We'll all pull together as a family (including siblings) and learn how to cope with this successfully."

Because children will have diabetes for life and because they need to learn from the beginning how to manage it, it is important that both parents agree to view the diabetes the same way and to treat the child consistently. Even if the two of you argue privately, you need to present a united front to your child so as not to send mixed messages about treatment and the emotional impact of the disease.

The way parents treat children should not change after the diagnosis. After all, they are still the same person, now needing sympathy, understanding, and skilled attention, as well as the love you have always shown.

Agnes is thirteen years old and has had diabetes since she was four. She still can't give herself an insulin injection and can manage to stick herself with the blood glucose lancet only every once in a while. Her parents do it the rest of the time and they always give her insulin injections. She has never slept overnight at a friend's house, and her parents do not permit her to go on school field trips.

Her father said she'll go to the community college nearby and live at home with her parents. Her parents think they are protecting Agnes, but in fact they are preventing her from learning to take care of herself and becoming an adult.

One way you can show that nothing essential has changed about the parent-child relationship is by maintaining discipline. It might appear almost cruel to punish children who have fallen ill with a serious disease, and it seems natural to let children do and have whatever they desire, but this is a mistake.

Withdrawing discipline is jarring, and the child may misinterpret it. For instance, if you have been honest about the fact that diabetes is serious but entirely controllable, the child could think, "They say this isn't that bad, but they're letting me do all the things I was never allowed to do before. That must mean they feel *really* sorry for me, so maybe I'm going to die. Why else would they be so lenient?"

This kind of thinking is scary for a child. Maintaining discipline and established limits demonstrates love and caring, and even a hint of the withdrawal of love at so crucial a time would be devastating. Setting limits and establishing good habits are preparation for the future. If these are ignored, children with diabetes could easily come to believe that they have no future.

This is not to say that there won't be changes in the way family members relate to one another; there will be. There will be jealousy, resentment, and perhaps more serious problems on the part of the diabetic child's siblings. It is not that they want diabetes, but being sick means that one gets a great deal of attention. Young children don't understand that this sudden diminution of attention away from them and onto a sibling has nothing to do with them and it is not the result of their behavior. All they see is their parents focusing a great deal on the sick child, and they get jealous and may begin to act out in inappropriate ways. On the other hand, they may be fearful they will "catch" diabetes from the sibling. They may be ridiculed and shunned at school, and their grades may drop.

So there may be a lot going on in your household for a while after the diagnosis. You're probably going to be busy, harried, worried, and scared. But you and your family do not have to go through this alone. There are a number of sources of help such as family therapists, school counselors, and all the health care providers mentioned in chapter 6. The important thing for you to remember is that, although your child's diabetes will last forever, the crisis mode that you may be functioning in at the beginning will not.

Learning about Diabetes

Parents' primary jobs are to learn enough about the disease in order to care for their children, keep them safe, and teach them how to grow up to be good diabetes managers.

How much knowledge is enough? That's hard to say. It's like asking how much education is enough. If you want to be a good car mechanic, you need to finish high school and then learn how to work on cars, either in an apprentice program or in a program with formal training. If you want to be a college professor, you probably need to go the whole route and earn a doctoral degree. If you want to be a secretary, you'd better learn how to spell and punctuate.

If you want to raise a healthy diabetic child who can control the physical aspects of the disease and learn to come to grips with the emotional ones, you need some basic facts. There are a number of ways you can do this:

- Read all you can on the subject. In addition to this book, you need to buy a few volumes that concentrate specifically on childhood diabetes. Keep them handy as references.
- Subscribe to magazines. The two best for you are *Countdown,* a publication of the Juvenile Diabetes Foundation, and *Diabetes Forecast,* published by the American Diabetes Association (see Resources).
- Join a support or self-help group that does more than hold discussions about emotions. While you will probably need a lot of emotional support at the beginning, you will also need something more: to learn as much as you can as quickly as you can. Therefore, a group that has speakers on a variety of topics is what you should look for. If you can't find one, ask your child's physician to put you in touch with other parents of diabetic children and form your own group.

- Join the Juvenile Diabetes Foundation. It can provide a lot of important and helpful information.

Giving a Child Insulin

Most children need at least two or three injections of insulin each day, usually short- and intermediate-acting. The dosing schedule will be prescribed by the physician and will be adjusted frequently as your child progresses through the four stages of Type I diabetes. In general though, children do best on a morning mixed dose of short- and intermediate-acting insulin a half hour before breakfast, a second injection of either a mixed dose or a dose of short-acting insulin a half hour before supper, and a third injection of intermediate-acting insulin at bedtime.

There are exceptions to this. For example, very young children who go to bed at six or seven in the evening usually can be controlled with a single mixed-dose injection in the morning.

The need to adjust the dose of insulin is based on blood glucose levels over a period of time, usually three days. An occasional high or low is nothing to be concerned about. It is most likely due to erratic eating or a change in the child's amount of physical activity. If, however, you begin to see a clear pattern indicating a permanent change in blood glucose, you need to call the doctor, who may change the dose. This is nothing to worry about, but it *is* one more thing your child will have to learn and get used to: the fact that diabetes is a dynamic disease—one's body responds to management in various ways depending on a number of external factors. Because children are such creatures of habit and routine, this "lesson" can be difficult and scary.

Meals and snacks should be eaten on a regular schedule, both to coordinate with the insulin and to teach the child good habits for the future. This is not as difficult as it seems. Breakfast is usually at the same time each school morning (weekend breakfasts can be delayed for a little while but no more than an hour), lunch at school is at a set time every day, and you are probably used to the family sitting down to supper at roughly the same time every evening. If this has not been the practice at your house, now would be a good time to begin the habit of family meals; they serve a far greater purpose than setting a routine for a diabetic child.

The Injection Process

You may have felt as though you were going to faint the first time you gave your child an insulin injection, and you may still be a little shaky. You may not believe this, but there will come a time, sooner than you think, when insulin injections will become so routine that you'll hardly realize that you're sticking a needle into your child.

Very few people already know how to give an injection, so it is extremely important that you learn from a professional: a nurse or a diabetes educator. If you are seeing a pediatric endocrinologist, most likely there will be someone on staff to help you. If not, you will probably be referred to such a person, who has experience in dealing with nervous parents. Ask as many questions as you need to when you are being taught (there is no such thing as a "dumb question" when you are dealing with your child's health), and don't hesitate to call when you have more questions. If you need another teaching session, ask for it.

The process of filling the syringe is exactly the same as it is for adults (see chapter 5), but there are a number of ways you can make the experience less painful and traumatic for your child:

- Until the child gets used to it and no longer thinks of an injection as painful, put an ice cube on the site for a few seconds. It will desensitize the skin and might even be fun for the child.
- Most of the "pain" associated with an injection isn't actually pain; it's fear, anxiety, and anticipation of pain. Therefore, if you present a calm, matter-of-fact demeanor and do not intimate that this is going to hurt, your child will quickly adopt your attitude.
- Let other family members give the injection once in a while. This serves two important functions: It keeps you from being the sole giver of needles, and it teaches others the skill.
- Try using some of the alternative insulin delivery systems, such as a pen injector or air jet infuser. Your child may think they're "cool," and in many cases they are easier to manipulate. You might also try an injection aid that fits over the end of the syringe (it hides the needle) and rests against the skin. It is designed to make certain that the angle of injection is correct, and is good for people who tend to be squeamish about injections. They are advertised in diabetes magazines and can be purchased through the mail.

- Use the shortest, finest gauge needles you can buy (the higher the number of the needle, the finer the gauge). This minimizes pain.
- Once the insulin has been drawn into the syringe, give the injection quickly. Don't diddle around with long, drawn-out preparations, and don't slide the needle in slowly. A quick stick is the least painful.

It is difficult to say at what age children can be taught to give themselves insulin injections; by nine or ten, they can do it if you or another adult supervises them, and some children can manage it even younger. By age twelve or thirteen, they should be able to be on their own with the injections—realizing, of course, that you will be there if they run into trouble. At whatever age you decide to teach the skill, it should be a shared responsibility for the first few weeks.

Teaching children how to measure the insulin, draw it up into the syringe, and insert the needle won't be entirely strange to them, of course, just as driving a car is not entirely strange to adolescents the first time they get behind the wheel. The experience is new, but much of the knowledge is already in place. As children watch their parents accelerate, steer, brake, and maneuver in traffic, so too they watch their parents test their blood glucose, calculate insulin dosage, and push the needle through the skin.

As with learning any new skill while a child is growing up, there will be periods of advance and backsliding. Some days a child will feel fiercely independent and will barely tolerate your presence in the room during the injection. Other days, you may be asked to do it. This back and forth is a natural process of growing up, and just because you have taught the technique does not mean that your child will get it right every time. This is why you need to supervise the process until you are absolutely certain it can be done alone.

Glucose Testing

As important as teaching children to give their own insulin is teaching them to understand the significance of self blood glucose monitoring and teaching them to use the monitor themselves.

Even though a finger prick is part of the test, it is much less complicated than giving an insulin injection, and children can be taught to do it themselves earlier than they are ready to give themselves injections. Most of them don't mind the finger stick because they don't have to jab a needle into themselves; it's spring loaded and automatic when a button is depressed. Moreover, a lot of kids think the monitor is "neat," and they like to show it off to their friends, even brag about it a little.

When the diabetes is first diagnosed, you and your child will have to test blood glucose fairly often, but after a few weeks it generally doesn't need to be done more than twice a day, which means that your child doesn't have to take the monitor to school. You need to keep a written record: time of day and the result. Once a week or every ten days, you should test blood glucose four times a day to be certain that everything is on track and that insulin injections and food intake remains in balance. And if the child has been especially active during the day, test blood glucose at bedtime. If it is low, a bedtime snack is in order.

When you teach blood glucose testing, do it one step at a time after your child has watched you for a while. Provide plenty of praise and encouragement, as you would when teaching any new skill, and when mistakes occur, don't scold, simply repeat the instruction.

If the result turns out to be higher or lower than normal, try not to be judgmental or punitive: "You must have eaten something you weren't supposed to," or "Have you been running around all afternoon when you were supposed to be studying for your history exam?" And don't freak out with worry (or if you absolutely have to, don't let your child know). It doesn't do any good: it won't change the read out on the blood glucose monitor, but it will create anger and resentment.

Rather, approach things from a problem solving point of view: "Let's give you an extra little jolt of insulin so we can get this number back down where it belongs," or "How about a half a chicken sandwich to tide you over till supper." If blood glucose is significantly elevated or depressed for three days running, the response should not be, "There's something really wrong with you. We'd better get you right to the doctor." Try instead, "I'm sure it's nothing serious, but let's just call Dr. Jones and see what he says about these numbers."

From the very beginning, always make sure that your child knows what the results of the blood glucose tests are—even a very young child, and even when you do all the testing. This accomplishes two things: It teaches awareness of what is happening with the diabetes and creates early training in responsibility for one's own care, and it fosters an open and honest attitude about the disease—and about your relationship with your child.

Most of the same things that affect adult blood glucose levels affect those of a child: illness, stress, more exercise than usual, inappropriate eating habits. It's up to you to find out what's been going on in your child's life when blood glucose is too high or too low for several tests in a row. When you find the cause, use it as a learning experience, not a punitive one.

Siblings should be a part of this enterprise as well. They are a part of the family, and childhood diabetes is most assuredly a family situation. They should know how to test their brother or sister's blood glucose (and to give an insulin injection) because one day they may have to do it and because it is part of the responsibility of helping to care for those we love.

Testing for Ketones

Ketone testing is done by dipping a test strip into urine, just as it is with adults. You should test for ketones when blood glucose is too high and/or at the first sign of illness and continue doing it until the child has recovered.

Boys can urinate into a disposable paper or plastic cup, and girls can be taught to hold a plastic cup against their vulva when they urinate. Eventually they will become adept at this. I know a little girl who can pee directly onto the strip. Most of the time she doesn't even get her hand wet, and says, "But I always wash my hands with soap and water anyway. Mommy taught me that safe is better than sorry."

If the test is positive for ketones, call the doctor immediately. Ketoacidosis is nothing to fool around with (see chapter 9).

14

The Future of Diabetes Treatment

The recent expansion of federal funding for diabetes research should help advance medical research programs now in progress. It is not impossible that within the next few decades there will be a cure for diabetes.

Living Transplants

One of the most promising areas of research is transplantation of living tissue from an individual who does not have diabetes to one who does. The most obvious choices are beta cells, islets of Langerhans, or a complete pancreas.

Rejection reaction is the major problem with transplantation of any cells, tissue, or organs. Heart and kidney transplant patients have to take immunosuppressive drugs for the rest of their lives in order to prevent their own immune systems from rejecting the transplanted organ. So must diabetics who receive transplants, and therein lies a serious stumbling block to successful cell transplantation: immunosuppressive drugs are highly toxic and cause serious side effects.

The type of transplant that carries the least risk of rejection is "pure" beta cells, that is, those that are not attached to any other tissue. However, pure beta cells are incredibly difficult to isolate in sufficient numbers needed for transplantation. If a person is given part of a pancreas, such as the islets of Langerhans, the rejection problems are the same as they are with a heart or kidney—unless the donor is an identical twin.

Islet Cells

Still, the most intensive transplantation research centers on islet cells. Scientists believe that such a transplant would be ideal because functional islets would restore normal insulin production. In theory, they would have to be implanted only once because islet cells survive for many years and carry within them the precursor cells needed to supply replacements for cells that die. The theory is workable, but the practice has proved difficult.

Researchers have obtained islet cells from laboratory rats and successfully transplanted them into animals of the same strain (genetically identical). The rats, which had been given diabetes artificially, received the cells, and their blood glucose levels returned to normal and stayed there. In other words, they were cured of diabetes.

This encouraged scientists to try the procedure in humans, but collecting islet cells from a human pancreas is far more difficult than doing so in a laboratory animal, primarily because of the number of cells involved. A human being requires about a million cells, but only about 400,000 can be collected using the procedure devised for rats.

Even when a method was developed to harvest enough cells, problems remained: First, the immune system would reject the cells, and immunosuppressive drugs have dangerous side effects, including cancer, kidney damage, and increased infection. Other problems included: clumping of islet cells with resultant clogging of the tubing used to infuse the cells into the recipient; destruction of islet cells during storage after they were harvested from the pancreas; and insufficient organ donors from whom to harvest islet cells.

Many of these problems have been diminished (rather than solved), and since 1990, about 145 people worldwide have received islet transplants from cadavers. In most cases, the cells have been unable to control blood glucose completely or have lost some of their activity after less than three years. Most of the reasons for failure stemmed from the original problems. Despite these setbacks, islet cell transplant research is in full swing, and eventually the procedure with human or pig islet cells will likely be used to treat, if not entirely cure, Type I diabetes.

Scientists are now engaged in studies to see if bone marrow infusions (transplants) given with islet cells from the same donor can eliminate the need for permanent immunosuppressive drugs. Since technology has enabled researchers to collect enough islet cells from a single donor pancreas rather than having to resort to multiple donors, giving bone marrow cells from that donor along with the islet cells may suppress the rejection reaction that has been so problematic. If successful, it could significantly change the course of treatment for Type I diabetics for two reasons: They would need only about a year of immunosuppressive therapy before being tapered off these potent drugs, and islet cells could be transplanted before a diabetic suffers kidney damage and requires a transplant of that organ.

Clinical trials will be limited initially to people with severe forms of Type I disease who have poorly controlled diabetes but have not yet developed significant complications. If successful, the trials will be expanded to include other Type I diabetics.

However, availability remains a serious problem; there will always be more people who need a pancreas than there are those willing to donate them. Moreover, research on the transplant of islet cells has slowed because of political pressure. A major source of islet cells for research has been fetal tissue, and antiabortion groups have been successful in establishing a government moratorium on such research. It is possible to do research on fetal tissue at private, nongovernmental institutions, but all major medical centers receive federal funding; therefore, they are not permitted to engage in research on fetal tissue.

Artificial Pancreas

An artificial pancreas, also called a closed-loop system, is a self-regulating device that contains all the elements of real beta cells. It controls blood glucose level with an electronic sensor that measures current glucose level, a pump to inject insulin, a reservoir to contain insulin, a small reservoir of glucose or glucagon to counteract hypoglycemia, and a power source to operate the system. In a way, it is a little like the currently available insulin pump, but it goes further. The insulin pump depends on the diabetic person to program it, and it does not measure blood glucose level. You have to do that yourself.

The artificial pancreas will not be available for many years because finding a material to house the internal glucose sensor without compromising accuracy has been impossible. Once this problem has been solved, and a fail-safe system devised, development will be relatively uncomplicated because miniaturization of electronic devices will make the entire apparatus practical.

There is a device now on the market called a Biostator, which can test and control blood glucose. It is worn outside the body attached by a catheter to a vein. About a half teaspoon of blood per hour, mixed with heparin to prevent clogging the catheter, is sent past a glucose sensor, which triggers the machine to release the proper amount of insulin or glucose through the catheter into the bloodstream.

The Biostator is useful in hospitals when patients are unconscious or on life support systems, but it is cumbersome and takes a great deal of skill to use properly. It is not appropriate for diabetics to use themselves.

Noninvasive Blood Glucose Monitoring

If you have ever had surgery, you probably remember a small device that was placed on your index finger. It is shaped like half a plastic clothespin and fits over both sides of the first joint and taped in place. This is called an oximeter and, without pricking your skin or inserting a needle, a beam of light close to the infrared spectrum passes through the finger and measures the amount of oxygen carried by the red blood cells. The oximeter is one of the many medical uses of space technology.

A similar device can be used to measure glucose, also without pricking the skin or inserting a needle. It is called a transducer. The machine is placed on the skin under the forearm, and through electronic signals, it measures the amount of glucose in tissue or blood. The technology was first developed by the agriculture industry to measure the amount of sugar in ripening potatoes and orchard fruit to determine optimal time for harvesting. The transducer is large and cumbersome and is now used only in physicians' offices. It's also very expensive.

Another device is the GlucoWatch, which is currently in the early phase of testing. It works by extracting glucose molecules through the skin with a low-level electric current. A disposable pad placed on the back of the watch collects glucose from fluid drawn through the skin.

Don't get excited about the imminent availability of a noninvasive glucose monitor; there have been too many insurmountable problems, and human testing is in the very earliest stages.

Alternate Methods of Insulin Delivery

No matter how accustomed diabetics are to giving themselves insulin injections, everyone would jump for joy at the prospect of taking insulin without jabbing it in with a needle. Several promising methods are now in the research stage.

Skin Patch

A skin patch like the ones used to deliver antismoking medications and seasickness preventives is under development. The problem is the size of the insulin molecule that has to cross the skin: about thirty times the size of the molecules of all drugs now administered by skin patch. One company, however, claims that it has solved the problem and is now conducting human trials.

The patch would be applied every day, and each one would deliver a constant low dose of insulin. The patch has six tabs that can be pulled off by the person wearing it if it is necessary to release extra doses of insulin. The company says that the price of the patch would be about the same as the cost of injecting insulin, including needles, syringes, and other supplies. A great deal more testing needs to be done, however, before the patch can be submitted to the Food and Drug Administration for approval.

Implantable Pump

Research on an implantable insulin pump has progressed steadily, although problems remain. There is more than one pump design, but they work in similar ways: the pump is implanted under the skin, and a catheter leads from it into the abdominal cavity. The pump releases a basal infusion of insulin in timed pulses, and bolus insulin doses can be given by means of an external telemetry unit.

After trials in dogs, scientists implanted the pump in eighteen human beings in 1986. Various adverse effects occurred: infection of the fibrous tissue that forms around the pump; electronic failure; and fibrous tissue blockage of the catheter leading from the pump into the abdominal cavity. Since then, more than four hundred people have received an implantable pump on an experimental basis in twenty medical centers across the United States.

The device has a number of advantages: It eliminates the need to change a catheter; there is no worry of incorrectly placed needles; an external pump does not have to be worn; and the danger of infection from handling the needle and catheter is removed. The major advantage, however, is the precision of insulin dosage with resultant excellent blood glucose control.

Disadvantages include problems with reliability and safety, the need for surgery, the possibility of catheter blockage, the need for very frequent blood glucose testing, and the cost.

Inhalation

Inhaling insulin is another possibility. Two methods are under study: nasal spray and aerosolized inhaler. Insulin is delivered even more rapidly from the mucous membranes inside the nose than when injected under the skin, but the fraction of the dose actually absorbed is much smaller—only about 10 to 20 percent. Insulin breathed in through an inhaler has the advantage of a larger surface from which to absorb it—lungs as opposed to the nose—but research on both methods is in only the early stages.

Oral Insulin Substitutes

An international research collaboration is now in the process of designing, synthesizing, and testing a new diabetes drug that can be taken as a pill to substitute for injected insulin. Researchers will use computer-assisted modeling to identify promising chemicals that mimic insulin.

Genetically engineered insulin already exists; this project will take the next step: making a synthetic drug that can be taken orally, absorbed into the bloodstream, and carried to cells without being destroyed. The research team will try to design a molecule that resembles part of the insulin hormone, which will fit into receptor molecules on the surface of cells the way insulin itself does.

Diabetes Prevention

In late 1996, the National Institutes of Health launched a nationwide clinical study to determine if taking a capsule of insulin crystals can prevent or delay Type I diabetes. The oral insulin test is the second phase of the Diabetes Prevention Trial, which is focusing on Type I and is designed for people at moderate risk of developing diabetes. Phase I, insulin injection intervention, was begun in early 1994 by the NIDDK and enrolls volunteers at high risk for developing diabetes.

Preliminary studies on animals have shown that it may be possible to prevent Type I diabetes with insulin. Scientists emphasize that insulin crystals cannot be used to treat diabetes because the body digests them, but they may stop the body's immune system from destroying insulin-producing cells. The process is called oral tolerization and will test whether one can alter the balance between protective and destructive immune system cells and halt the destructive process.

Researchers at ten centers across the country (and 350 recruitment offices) are screening people for the study. Volunteers must have a relative with Type I diabetes and be age three to forty-five years. Such people can call 800-425-8361 for eligibility information.

Genetic Research

Although there are many contributing factors, diabetes is basically a genetic disease. It has always been thought to run in families, but with establishment of the Human Biological Data Interchange (HBDI), that supposition has now been positively demonstrated. The HBDI, based in Philadelphia, looks for families with diabetic children and collects immortal cell lines for diabetes researchers. Immortal cells are those taken from blood and allowed to replicate without limit in a laboratory, as a continuous source of DNA. About six thousand families consisting of seventy-five thousand people are now in the HBDI database, which is accessible to researchers around the world. All blood samples taken from family members are typed for HLA, the place on a chromosome that determines most of a person's susceptibility to Type I diabetes.

Scientists have known for a long time that Type I diabetes is an autoimmune disease; that is, one's own immune system destroys beta cells in the pancreas. At the same time, it is a multifactorial disease, which means that a number of factors contribute to it, only one of which is inheritance. However, diabetes does not follow the usual laws of inherited diseases, such as occurs in Huntington's disease, Tay-Sachs disease, sickle cell anemia, and cystic fibrosis. In these diseases, it is certain that if one or both parents carry the gene for a disease, children will have a specific statistical risk of also having the disease.

Scientists have known that the genetic region known as HLA figured strongly in autoimmune diseases, but they didn't know how. It has now been discovered that the HLA region of chromosome six and chromosome eleven contain variations that influence susceptibility to Type I diabetes.

Moreover, familial diabetes is a polygenic disorder; that is, although it is associated with genetic traits, those traits differ from family to family. This means that the search for genes responsible for susceptibility to diabetes on the entire human genome (the complete "library" of hereditary instructions contained in all forty-six human chromosomes) could take decades and cost billions of dollars.

But with the HBDI, that search can be shortened and simplified, although it is by no means an easy task. With cell samples from all members of a family, family trees, which show relationships and the presence or absence of diabetes in each member, are now available for study. In addition, a continuous supply of cells from those families can be used for study. In fact, the study of these six thousand families and their cells is the sole occupation of a significant number of diabetes researchers. It has become one of the most important areas of diabetes research.

Glossary

Adult-onset diabetes—The former term for Type II diabetes.

Adverse effect—A harmful result that usually refers to negative effects of medications.

Albuminuria—Having more than the normal amount of a protein called albumin in the urine; this may be a sign of kidney disease and usually occurs in people who have had diabetes for a long time.

Alpha cell—A type of cell in the pancreas that makes and releases a hormone called glucagon, which raises blood glucose level.

Amino acid—The building block of proteins, which constitute the body's cells. Insulin is composed of fifty-one amino acids.

Angiopathy—A disease of the blood vessels. There are two types: macroangiopathy affects large vessels, and microangiopathy affects small vessels.

Antidiabetic agent—A substance that helps a person with diabetes control blood glucose levels; also called oral hypoglycemic agent.

Arteriosclerosis—A group of diseases in which the walls of the arteries thicken and harden.

Artery—A blood vessel that carries blood from the heart to other parts of the body.

Artificial pancreas—A machine used in hospitals to constantly measure blood glucose and, in response, release the correct amount of insulin.

Aspartame—An artificial, noncaloric sweetener.

Autoimmune disease—A disorder of the body's immune system in which it mistakenly attacks and destroys body tissue that it believes to be foreign, for example insulin-dependent diabetes.

Autonomic neuropathy—A disease of the nerves, which are not under conscious control, that affects mostly internal organs such as the bladder, cardiovascular system, digestive tract, and genital organs.

Background retinopathy—The early stages of diabetic retinopathy (also called nonproliferative retinopathy), which usually does not impair vision.

Beta cell—A cell in the pancreas that makes and releases insulin.

Biosynthetic human insulin—Artificial human insulin that is genetically identical to natural insulin.

Biphasic insulin—A combination of intermediate- and fast-acting insulin, also called a mixed dose.

Blood glucose—The amount of glucose in the bloodstream.

Blood glucose monitor (meter)—A machine, designed to be used by individuals at home, that tests the amount of glucose in the blood.

Blood pressure—The force of the blood on the walls of arteries. Two levels of blood pressure are measured: systolic pressure (the upper number), which occurs each time the heart pushes blood into the vessels, and diastolic pressure (the lower number), which occurs when the heart rests.

Blood urea nitrogen (BUN)—A waste product of the kidneys. Elevated BUN may indicate early kidney disease.

Bolus—An extra boost of insulin given to cover an expected rise in blood glucose, such as that which occurs after eating.

Brittle diabetes—A term used when the blood glucose level often swings quickly from high to low; also called labile or unstable diabetes.

Bronze diabetes—A genetic disease of the liver in which the body takes in too much iron from food; also called hemochromatosis.

Capillary—The smallest of the body's blood vessels through which glucose passes into cells.

Carbohydrate—One of the three main classes of food, composed mainly of sugar and starch, which is eventually broken down into glucose and used for energy.

Cardiovascular—Something pertaining to the heart and blood vessels.

Cataract—The clouding of the lens of the eye.

Certified diabetes educator (C.D.E.)—A health care professional certified by the American Association of Diabetes Educators to teach people with diabetes how to manage their disease.

Charcot foot—A condition associated with diabetic neuropathy that results in destruction of joints and soft tissue; also called Charcot's joint or neuropathic arthropathy.

Cholesterol—A fat-like substance found in blood, liver, brain, and other tissues. If too much cholesterol builds up in artery walls, the flow of blood may be blocked to a vital organ such as the heart or brain.

Chronic—Present over a long period of time; for example, diabetes as a chronic disease.

Clinical trial—A scientifically controlled study carried out in human beings to test safety and efficacy of a new treatment.

Coma—A deep unconsciousness. Diabetic coma is a severe emergency because blood glucose is dangerously low or high.

Congenital defects—Problems or conditions present at birth.

Congestive heart failure—Loss of pumping power of the heart, resulting in excessive fluids collecting in the body.

Contraindication—A condition under which a treatment or medication should not be instituted.

Coxsackie B4 virus—A virus that damages beta cells of the pancreas, which may be a contributory factor in insulin-dependent diabetes.

C-peptide—A substances the pancreas releases into the bloodstream in amounts equal to insulin. A test of the C-peptide level will show how much insulin the body is making.

Dawn phenomenon—The sudden rise in blood glucose level in the early morning hours, usually seen in insulin-dependent diabetes.

Dehydration—The excessive loss of body water, sometimes caused by very high blood glucose.

Delta cell—A cell in the pancreas that makes and releases somatostatin, a hormone believed to control how beta cells make and release insulin and how alpha cells make and release glucagon.

Dextrose—A simple sugar found in the blood; also called glucose.

Diabetes control and complications trial (DCCT)— A ten-year study (1983–1993) funded by the National Institute of Diabetes and Digestive and Kidney Diseases to assess the effects of intensive therapy on long-term complications of diabetes.

Diabetes insipidus—A disease of the pituitary gland or kidney. The cause and treatment are different from those of diabetes mellitus.

Diabetic retinopathy—A disease of the small blood vessels of the retina of the eye, which causes blurry vision. If left untreated and the disease progresses, vision can be severely affected.

Dietician—An expert in nutrition who can help devise a food plan; also called nutritionist.

Dilated pupil examination—Use of special drops to enlarge the pupils of the eyes in order to view the back of the eye, especially blood vessels.

Diuretic—A drug that increases the flow of urine.

Edema—Swelling or puffiness in a part of the body, such as the ankles, due to a collection of water and other fluids.

Endocrine glands—Glands, such as the pancreas, that release hormones into the bloodstream.

Endocrinologist—A physician who specializes in treating diseases of endocrine glands, such as diabetes.

Enzyme—A type of protein that helps body chemistry work better and more quickly. Each enzyme usually has only one function, such as transforming starch into glucose.

Epinephrine—A secretion of the adrenal glands (located above each kidney) that helps the liver release glucose and limits release of insulin; also called adrenaline.

Euglycemia—Normal blood glucose.

Exchange list—The grouping of foods by type to give people on special diets the opportunity to substitute one food for another of the same type. There are six groups: starch/bread, meat, vegetables, fruit, milk, and fats.

Fasting blood glucose—Testing blood glucose in the morning when nothing has been eaten for ten to twelve hours prior.

Fats—One of the three main classes of foods and a source of energy. In food there are two types of fat: saturated fats are solid at room temperature and are found mainly in animal products, and unsaturated fats are liquid at room temperature and consist mainly of plant oils.

Fiber—A food substance found in plants that helps in the digestive process and that is believed to lower cholesterol and help control blood glucose.

Fractional urine—A twenty-four hour collection of urine, also called block urine.

Fructose—A type of sugar found in many fruits and vegetables and in honey.

Galactose—A type of sugar found in milk products and sugar beets.

Gestational diabetes—A type of diabetes that occurs during pregnancy and almost always disappears after delivery.

Glaucoma—An eye disease associated with increased pressure inside the eyeball. It can damage the optic nerve and cause impaired vision and blindness.

Glucagon—A hormone that raises the level of blood glucose. An injectable form is sometimes used to treat insulin shock.

Glucose—A simple sugar found in the blood, which is the body's main source of energy; also called dextrose.

Glucose tolerance test—A succession of three blood samples, taken after drinking liquid glucose, to see how well the body deals with glucose in the blood over a period of time.

Glycemic response—The effect of different foods on blood glucose.

Glycogen—A substance composed of sugars, which is stored in the liver and muscles, that releases glucose into the blood when needed by cells.

Glycosuria—The presence of glucose in the urine.

Glycosylated hemoglobin test—A blood test that measures average blood glucose for the past three months; also called glycohemoglobin and hemoglobin A1C, which is the substance of red blood cells that sometimes joins with glucose. Because glucose stays attached for the life of the cell (about three months), hemoglobin A1C shows average glucose for that period of time.

Gram—A unit of weight in the metric system. There are twenty-eight grams in an ounce.

High blood pressure (hypertension)—A condition in which blood flows through the vessels at greater than normal force, which puts a strain on the heart and increases the risk of heart attack, stroke, and kidney problems.

Hormone—A chemical released by special cells to tell other cells what to do, for instance when the hormone insulin tells cells to use glucose.

Human insulin—Artificial insulin similar to that produced by the human body.

Hyperglycemia—Elevated blood glucose, a sign that diabetes is out of control.

Hyperinsulinism—An elevated level of insulin in the blood.

Hypoglycemia—Too little blood glucose, a sign that diabetes is out of control.

Hypotension—Low blood pressure or a sudden drop in blood pressure.

Implantable insulin pump—Small pump placed inside the body that delivers insulin in response to telemetric commands from a hand-held device.

Injection site rotation—Changing the places on the body where one injects insulin, which prevents lumps or small dents from forming in the skin.

Insulin—A hormone, made in and released from beta cells in the pancreas, that helps the body use glucose.

Insulin antagonist—Something that opposes or fights the action of insulin, such as glucagon.

Insulin binding—When insulin attaches itself to something else, for example, to the outer part of a cell, in response to the cell's need for energy.

Insulin pump—A device that delivers a continuous supply of insulin into the body. Insulin flows from the pump through a plastic tube connected to a needle inserted into the body.

Insulin reaction—Reaction to too large an injection of insulin, too little food consumed, or exercise without sufficient food.

Insulin receptor—The area on the outer part of a cell that allows the cell to bind with insulin in the blood.

Insulin resistance—Nonresponse or poor response of the body to the action of the body's own insulin.

Insulin shock—A severe condition occasioned by a rapid drop of blood glucose.

Intensive management—A treatment of insulin-dependent diabetes in which the main objective is to keep blood glucose levels as close to a normal range as possible; also called tight control.

Islet cell transplantation—Moving groups of beta cells from a donor pancreas into a person whose pancreas has stopped producing insulin.

Islets of Langerhans—Groups of cells in the pancreas that make and secrete insulin.

Ketoacidosis—Severe out-of-control diabetes that occurs when blood glucose is too high, during which the body starts using stored fat for energy and ketones build up in the blood.

Ketones—Chemicals formed in the blood when the body uses fat instead of glucose for energy. If ketones form, it usually means that cells do not have enough insulin or cannot use the insulin that is in the bloodstream. Ketones pass through the body into the urine and can poison and even kill cells.

Ketonuria—The presence of ketones in the urine, which is a warning sign of diabetic ketoacidosis.

Lactose—A type of sugar found in milk and milk products.

Lipid—Body fat.

Macrosomia—Abnormally large. In terms of diabetes, it refers to abnormally large babies (more than nine pounds) delivered by diabetic women.

Macrovascular disease—A disease of the large blood vessels, usually seen in long-term diabetics as a result of poor glucose control.

Macular edema—Edema in the macula, an area near the center of the retina of the eye responsible for fine or reading vision.

Metabolism—The way cells chemically change food to keep the body alive. It is a two-part process: catabolism, in which the body uses food for energy; and anabolism, in which the body uses food to build or repair cells.

Microaneurysm—A small swelling on the side of tiny blood vessels, often in the eyes of diabetics, that may break and bleed into nearby tissue.

Microvascular disease—A disease of the small blood vessels, usually seen in long-term diabetics as a result of poor glucose control.

Mixed dose—Combining two kinds of insulin in one injection; also called a combination dose.

National Institute of Diabetes and Digestive and Kidney Diseases (NIDDK)—One of the institutes that comprise the National Institutes of Health, an agency of the U.S. Public Health Service.

Nephropathy—Disease of the kidneys caused by damage to the small vessels or to the units in the kidneys that clean the blood.

Neuropathy—A disease of the nervous system.

Noninvasive blood glucose monitoring—Measuring blood glucose without having to prick the skin to obtain a drop of blood.

Nutrition—The process by which the body draws nutrients from food and uses them to make or repair cells.

Ophthalmologist—A physician who specializes in eyes.

Optometrist—A person trained to test eyes and detect and treat eye problems by prescribing and adapting corrective lenses and other devices; not a physician.

Oral hypoglycemic agent—A pill or capsule that lowers the level of blood glucose.

Pancreas—The organ behind the lower part of the stomach that contains the cells that make insulin.

Pancreas transplant—Surgically replacing the pancreas of a diabetic with either the healthy pancreas of a cadaver donor or with half the pancreas of a living relative. This procedure is done only on insulin-dependent diabetics with severe complications.

Pancreatitis—Inflammation of the pancreas.

Periodontal disease—Damage to the gums.

Peripheral neuropathy—Nerve damage affecting the hands, arms, feet, and legs, which causes pain, tingling, or numbness.

Peripheral vascular disease—A disease in the large blood vessels of the arms, legs, and feet, usually seen in long-term diabetics.

Podiatrist—A doctor who treats and takes care of feet; not a physician.

Polydipsia—A great thirst that lasts for long periods of time.

Polyphagia—Great hunger.

Postprandial blood glucose—Blood tested one to two hours after eating.

Preeclampsia—A condition, frequently seen in gestational diabetes, in the late stages of pregnancy characterized by high blood pressure and swelling of the feet and ankles.

Proinsulin—A substance originating from the pancreas that is then made into insulin. When insulin is purified from beef or pork, all the proinsulin is not removed, which can cause a person taking the insulin to break out in a rash or resist the insulin.

Proliferative retinopathy—A disease of the small blood vessels of the retina of the eye; also called diabetic retinopathy.

Protein—One of the three main classes of food, made of amino acids, also called the building blocks of the cells.

Purified insulin—Insulin with low levels of impure proinsulin, thought to minimize allergic and other untoward reactions.

Reagent—Chemically treated strips or tablets used to test the level of glucose in blood or urine.

Rebound—A swing to a too-high level of glucose in the blood after a too-low level; also called Somogyi effect.

Receptors—Areas on the outer part of a cell that allow the cell to bind with insulin.

Retina—The center part of the back lining of the eye that senses light.

Risk factor—Anything that increases the chance that one will get a disease; for example, being overweight is a risk factor for Type II diabetes.

Saccharin—A noncaloric artificial sweetener.

Secondary diabetes—Diabetes as a result of another disease or because of taking certain drugs or chemicals.

Sliding scale—Adjusting insulin on the basis of blood glucose tests, meals, and activity levels.

Somatostatin—A hormone made by delta cells of the pancreas, which may control how the body secretes insulin and glucagon.

Spilling point—When blood has too much of a substance such as glucose and the kidneys allow the excess to spill over into the urine; also called renal threshold.

Split dose—The division of a prescribed daily dose of insulin into two or more injections over the course of a day; also called multiple injections.

Subcutaneous injection—Putting a fluid such as insulin into the tissue under the skin with a needle and syringe.

Sucrose—Table sugar, which the body must break down into a simpler form before the blood can absorb it.

Syringe—A hollow glass or plastic tube, to which a needle is attached, used to inject medications.

Toxemia of pregnancy—A condition in which poisons such as the body's own waste products build up and may harm both pregnant woman and fetus.

Type I diabetes—Insulin-dependent diabetes.

Type II diabetes—Non-insulin-dependent diabetes.

Unit of insulin—The basic measure of insulin. U-100 insulin contains one hundred units of insulin per milliliter (also called cubic centimeter) of solution.

Urea—One of the chief waste products of the body, which is excreted in the urine.

Urine testing—Checking urine with reagents to determine if it contains glucose and ketones.

Vaginitis—A vaginal infection usually caused by a fungus, seen frequently in women with diabetes.

Vascular—Relating to blood vessels.

Vein—A blood vessel that carries blood to the heart.

American Diabetes Association Guidelines

The recently revised American Diabetes Association (ADA) guidelines (which were developed in cooperation with the American Dietetic Association) for the way diabetics should eat are nothing more than a guide to sensible eating for everyone. There is nothing fancy, nothing arcane, nothing "scientific," and nothing weird. If you've been eating healthily, you won't have to learn a whole new way of cooking and eating.

The guidelines cover how many grams of carbohydrate you can eat in a day to keep your blood glucose normal (this will vary from person to person—within a certain range), how many grams of fat you should limit yourself to, how to adjust your meals to exercise and medication, how many total calories you can eat per day to lose weight and maintain the loss, and how to manage food if you are ill.

Perhaps the best and most surprising statement from the ADA is: "Scientific evidence has shown that the use of sucrose (table sugar) as part of the meal plan does not impair blood glucose control in individuals with Type I or Type II diabetes."

This doesn't mean you can eat as many chocolate chip cookies as you want. What it does mean is that a sparing amount of sugar is part of a well-balanced diet, as long as it is eaten with other foods in place of other carbohydrates (remember, you need to count the total amount of carbohydrates in your meal plan). A snack that consists of only sugar can send blood glucose levels soaring.

In general, every day you should eat:

- Three to four servings each of fruit and vegetables (twenty to thirty-five grams of fiber)
- Three servings of foods from the bread, cereal, rice, and pasta group
- Two to three servings of food from the meat, poultry, fish, dry beans, eggs, and nuts group (10–20 percent of daily caloric intake should be from protein)
- Two to three servings from the dairy products group
- Only sparing intake of fats, oils, and sweets (no more than 30 percent of total daily calories)
- No more than 3,000 mg of sodium (2,400 mg for people with hypertension)

You will notice that this recommendation is almost the same as the U.S. Department of Health and Human Services food pyramid. The major exception is that the ADA guidelines suggest less food from the bread-pasta group.

In addition, the ADA suggests that instead of eating three square meals a day, a habit instilled in most Americans, you ought to try the "grazing" approach: eating five or six smaller meals throughout the day. This is not as difficult as it seems. Even if you are out of the house at work all day, you can do the following: eat breakfast at home; eat a small, late lunch; and in between the two, have a mini-meal on your morning break. Have another snack in late afternoon, eat a late supper at home, and then eat something before bedtime.

Since you need to lose weight and because everyone requires fewer calories as we age (because metabolism slows down about 2 percent a year), the ADA guidelines emphasize counting calories. One easy way to consume fewer calories without making a dent in the quality and palatability of your diet is to decrease the size of each portion of potentially high-calorie foods by about a third. Also, if you exercise within an hour of eating, when your metabolism is highest, you will burn more calories for the same amount of effort.

The ADA recommends that every diabetic create a meal plan in individual consultation with a registered dietician, and it suggests that the meal plan be tailored to the type of diabetes, the method of treatment, and whether you have a weight or other health problem. This is good advice, but it may not be practical for everyone. Some people do not have access to a dietician, some can't afford it if their health insurance policy won't reimburse for a dietician's services, and some people just won't bother. So you need to know how to make your own meal plan. It's not difficult. General guidelines are as follows:

- The total amount of carbohydrates consumed is the factor that influences blood glucose, not the food source of the carbohydrate.
- Count carbohydrates. All carbohydrates, regardless of the source, have four calories per gram.
- Type I diabetics and others on insulin should make every effort to eat at the same times every day, and the amount and types of food eaten at each meal should be about the same from day to day. This is important because food is coordinated with insulin injections.
- Review your meal plan periodically with your physician, diabetes educator, or dietician. Various circumstances may necessitate changes.

If you want a copy of the ADA guidelines, call the Order Fulfillment Department at 800-232-3472 and ask for a copy.

Exchange Groups

Exchange groups are exactly what they sound like: suggestions for substituting one food of a similar type for another. This is the mechanism used to create flexibility in your diabetic food plan. There are six basic groups into which all food is divided: milk, vegetable, fruit, bread/starch, meat, and fat.

Most diabetic exchange plans will specify the number of portions from each group of foods that you should eat at each meal. A portion (or choice as it is sometimes called) is a measured amount of food containing a certain amount of carbohydrate, protein, and fat. Each portion contains a certain number of calories and grams of fat.

The type and number of choices you will have depend on the number of calories you should eat in a day, anywhere from 1,200 to 2,500, depending on your physical activity and the amount of weight you need to lose.

Before you throw up your hands and tell yourself that this is much too restrictive and complicated, read on. A diabetic food plan (the same as an exchange meal plan) is, it's true, more restrictive than eating anything you want, whenever you want, in any amount you please. But a healthy person shouldn't be doing that anyway. You must follow other rules and guidelines in other spheres of your life: obeying speed limits and stopping at red lights, setting your alarm and hauling yourself out of bed to get to work on time even when you don't want to, refraining from talking and fooling around when you're at the theater or in church. Life is full of rules and social conventions. Think of a diabetic food plan as just another one. Moreover, the restrictions are not onerous. There is a tremendous amount of flexibility in a diabetic food plan.

Also, it's not complicated at all. You already know the food pyramid, you know what fruits and vegetables and meats are. All you have to do is fit them together in a pattern, which you've been doing anyway. No one eats a meal of all bananas or lives on nothing but chicken salad for two days. And even though it sounds good, few adults would eat nothing but sweets or fat-laden foods. Over the course of a day or two, people naturally gravitate toward a balanced and varied diet.

Developing and using a meal involves a few uncomplicated steps. First, learn the groups and the foods they contain. This may mean carrying a "cheat sheet" around with you for a while (a chart on which foods are listed according to group, or a photocopy of the following few pages), but soon you'll find that you can make choices and substitutions almost without thinking about it.

Second, plan your day. Know beforehand what you will eat and approximately when you will eat it, and try to eat each meal at about the same time each day. This is particularly important for Type I diabetics. Third, teach yourself which exchanges are permissible and which you should make as seldom as possible. In general, exchanges among foods in a group are okay, whereas exchanges between groups are not. For example, you could have a chicken sandwich for lunch instead of cold rice salad with sliced chicken, or vice versa. But chicken, even if it's a skinless breast grilled with no fat, is not a substitute for a serving of vegetable. The nutrients are not the same.

Starch/Bread

Each item on this list contains approximately fifteen grams of carbohydrate, three grams of protein, a trace of fat, and eighty calories.

Cereals/Grains/Pasta	**Bread**
Bran cereal, concentrated ⅓ cup	Bagel ½
Bran cereal, flaked ½ cup	Bread sticks ⅔ oz
Bulgur, cooked ½ cup	Croutons 1 cup
Cereals, cooked ½ cup	English muffin ½
Cornmeal, dry 2½ tb	Hot dog bun ½
Grape Nuts 3 tb	Hamburger bun ½
Grits, cooked ½ cup	Pita, 6-inch, ½
Other, unsweetened ¾ cup	Plain roll 1 oz
Pasta, cooked ½ cup	Raisin 1 slice
Puffed cereal 1½ cups	Rye 1 slice
Rice, cooked ⅓ cup	Pumpernickel 1 slice
Shredded wheat ½ cup	Tortilla, 6-inch, 1
Wheat germ 3 tb	White 1 slice
	Whole wheat 1 slice

Dried Beans/Peas/Lentils	**Crackers/Snacks**
Beans, peas, cooked ⅓ cup	Animal crackers 8
Lentils, cooked ⅓ cup	Graham crackers 3
Baked beans ¼ cup	Matzo ¾ oz
	Melba toast 5 sl
	Oyster crackers 2–4
	Popcorn, plain 3 cups
	Pretzels ¾ oz
	Rye crisps 4
	Saltines 6
	Whole wheat crackers ¾ oz

Starchy Vegetables (Prepared with Fat)	Starchy Foods (Prepared with Fat)
Corn ½ cup	Biscuit, 2½-inch, 1
Corn on the cob 1	Chinese noodles ½ cup
Lima beans ½ cup	Corn bread 2 oz
Peas ½ cup	Butter cracker 6
Plantain ½ cup	French fries 10
Potato, baked 1	Muffin, small, plain, 1
Potato, mashed ½ cup	Pancake, 4-inch, 2
Squash, winter ¾ cup	Stuffing, bread ¼ cup
Yam ⅓ cup	Taco shells, 6-inch, 2
	Waffle, 4½-inch, 1

Meat

Each serving on this list contains about seven grams of protein, and the amount of fat and number of calories vary: three grams of fat and fifty-five calories for lean meat; five grams of fat and seventy-five calories for medium-fat meat; and eight grams of fat and one hundred calories for high-fat meat.

Lean Meat	Medium-Fat Meat	High-Fat Meat
Beef, USDA Good, Choice 1 oz	Ground beef 1 oz	Beef, USDA Prime 1 oz
Pork, tenderloin 1 oz	Rib steak 1 oz	Spareribs 1 oz
Canadian bacon 1 oz	Porterhouse 1 oz	Pork sausage 1 oz
Veal 1 oz	Meat loaf 1 oz	Lamb, ground 1 oz
Poultry, skinless 1 oz	Pork chops 1 oz	Fish, fried 1 oz
Fish 1 oz	Lamb 1 oz	Lunch meat 1 oz
Shellfish 2 oz	Veal cutlet 1 oz	Hot dog 1
Wild game 1 oz	Poultry, skin 1 oz	

	Ground turkey 1 oz	
	Tuna, canned 1/4 cup	
	Salmon, canned 1/4 cup	

Vegetables

Each serving on this list contains about five grams of carbohydrate, two grams of protein, and twenty-five calories. Most vegetables contain two to three grams of fiber. The serving size for vegetables is one-half cup of cooked vegetables or vegetable juice and one cup of raw.

Vegetables	
Artichoke (one-half medium)	Mushrooms
Asparagus	Okra
Beans (green, wax, Italian)	Onions
Bean sprouts	Pea pods
Beets	Peppers (green)
Broccoli	Rutabaga
Brussels sprouts	Sauerkraut
Cabbage	Spinach
Carrots	Summer squash
Cauliflower	Tomato
Eggplant	Turnips
Greens (collard, mustard, turnip)	Water chestnuts
Kohlrabi	Zucchini
Leeks	

Fruit

Each item on this list contains about fifteen grams of carbohydrate and sixty calories. Fresh, frozen, and dried fruits have about two grams of fiber.

Fresh, Frozen, and Unsweetened Canned Fruit		
Apple, 2-inch, 1	Applesauce ½ cup	Apricots, canned ½ cup
Banana, 9-inch, ½	Blackberries ¾ cup	Blueberries ¾ cup
Cantaloupe, 5-inch, ⅓	Cherries, fresh 12	Cherries, canned ½ cup
Figs 2	Fruit cocktail, canned ½ cup	Grapefruit ½
Grapes 15	Honeydew melon 1⅛	Kiwi 1
Mandarin oranges ¾ cup	Mango ½	Nectarine 1
Orange 1	Papaya 1 cup	Peach, fresh 1
Peaches, canned 1 cup	Pear, fresh 1	Pears, canned ½ cup
Persimmons 2	Pineapple, raw ¾ cup	Pineapple, canned ⅓ cup
Plums 2	Pomegranate ½	Raspberries 1 cup
Strawberries 1¼ cups	Tangerine 2	Watermelon, cubed 1¼ cups

Dried Fruit	Fruit Juice
Apples 4 rings	Apple/cider ½ cup
Apricots 7 halves	Cranberry ⅓ cup
Dates 2½	Grapefruit ½ cup
Figs 1½	Grape ⅓ cup
Prunes 3	Orange ½ cup
Raisins 2 tb	Pineapple ½ cup
	Prune ⅓ cup

Milk

Each serving of milk or milk products contains about twelve grams of carbohydrate and eight grams of protein. The amount of fat is measured in percent of butterfat, and calories vary. The list is divided into three parts; one serving of each provides the following:

	Carbohydrate (gr)	Protein (gr)	Fat (gr)	Calories
Skim milk	12	8	trace	90
Low-fat milk	12	8	5	140
Whole milk	12	8	8	160

A serving size of skim and very low-fat milk is one cup. For evaporated skim milk, a serving is one-half cup, for dry nonfat milk, it's one-third cup, and for plain yogurt, eight ounces. For low-fat and whole milk (2 percent), a serving size is one cup, and for evaporated milk, it's one-half cup.

Fats

Each serving size on the fat list contains about five grams of fat and forty-five calories.

Avocado 1/8	Margarine 1 tsp
Margarine, diet 1 tb	Mayonnaise 1 tsp
Mayonnaise, low-cal 1 tb	Almonds, dry roasted 6
Cashews, dry roasted 1 tb	Pecans 2
Peanuts 10–20	Walnuts 2 whole
Seeds, no shells 1 tb	Pumpkin seeds 2 tsp
Oils 1 tsp	Olives 5–10
Salad dressing, mayonnaise 2 tsp	Salad dressing, regular 1 tb
Salad dressing, low-cal 2 tb	Chitterlings 1/2 oz
Coconut, shredded 2 tb	Coffee whitener, liquid 2 tb
Coffee whitener, powder 4 tsp	Cream, light 2 tb
Cream, heavy 1 tb	Sour cream 2 tb
Cream cheese 1 tb	Salt pork 1/4 oz
Butter 1 tsp	Bacon 1 slice

Free Foods

Foods on this list contain fewer than twenty calories per serving. You can eat as much as you want except where a serving size is noted when you can eat two or three servings a day.

Drinks	**Unsweetened Fruit**
Bullion or broth	Cranberries ½ cup
Sugar-free soda	Rhubarb ½ cup
Seltzer water (club soda)	
Cocoa powder, unsweetened 1 tb	
Coffee and tea	
Drink mixes, sugar free	
Tonic water, sugar free	

Vegetables (raw, 1 cup)	**Salad Greens**
Cabbage	Celery
Chinese cabbage	Escarole
Endive	Cucumber
Lettuce	Romaine
Green onion	Hot peppers
Spinach	Radishes
Mushrooms	
Zucchini	

Sweets (sugar free)	**Condiments**
Candy	Catsup 1 tb
Gelatin	Horseradish
Chewing gum	Mustard
Jam/jelly	Pickles
Pancake syrup	Taco sauce 1 tb
Sugar substitutes	Vinegar
Whipped topping 2 tb	

Seasonings

Basil	Celery seed
Cinnamon	Chili powder
Chives	Curry
Dill	Garlic
Flavoring extracts (vanilla, almond, lemon, etc.)	Herbs
Garlic powder	Lemon and lemon juice
Hot pepper sauce	Mint
Lime and lime juice	Oregano
Onion powder	Pepper
Paprika	Spices
Pimento	Cooking wine ¼ cup
Soy sauce	Worcestershire sauce

Resources

American Amputee Foundation
P.O. Box 250218
Little Rock, AR 72225
501-666-2523

American Association of Diabetes Educators
444 North Michigan Avenue, Suite 1240
Chicago, IL 60611
800-338-3633

American Board of Medical Specialties
47 Perimeter Center East, Suite 500
Atlanta, GA 30346
800-776-2378 or 770-551-5936

American Council of the Blind
1155 15 Street, N.W., Suite 720
Washington, DC 20005
800-424-8666 or 202-467-5081

American Diabetes Association
National Service Center
1600 Duke Street
Alexandria, VA 22314
800-ADA-DISC

American Dietetic Association
430 North Michigan Avenue
Chicago, IL 60611
800-877-1600

DEED (Diabetics Educating and Empowering Diabetics)
301-972-0617

Equal Employment Opportunity Commission
1801 L Street, N.W.
Washington, DC 10507
800-669-4000 or 800-669-6820
800-669-3362 for Americans with Disabilities Act publications

Impotence Institute of America
10400 Little Patuxent Parkway, Suite 485
Columbia, MD 21044
800-669-1603 or 410-715-9609

International Diabetes Center
3800 Park Nicollet Boulevard
St. Louis Park, MN 55416
612-983-3393

Joslin Diabetes Center
1 Joslin Place
Boston, MA 02215
617-732-2440

Juvenile Diabetes Foundation
432 Park Avenue South
New York, NY 20026
212-889-7575

Medic Alert Foundation (for ID bracelets)
P.O. Box 1009
Turlock, CA 95381-1009
800-432-5378

National Diabetes Information Clearinghouse
Box NDIC

Bethesda, MD 20892
301-468-2162

National Kidney Foundation
30 East 33 Street
New York, NY 10016
800-622-9010 or 212-689-9261

Social Security Administration
800-772-1213; or 800-638-6833 (Medicare Hotline)
U.S. Government Printing Office
Superintendent of Documents
Washington DC 20402-9328
(Free copy of "Nutritive Value of Foods")

On the Internet:
American Association of Clinical Endocrinologists
http://www.aace.com

American Association of Diabetes Educators
http://www.AADEnet.org

American Diabetes Association
http://www.diabetes.org

American Dietetic Association
http://www.eatright.org

Brigham and Women's Hospital, Boston, Arturo Rolla, M.D.
world.e.std.com

Canadian Diabetes Association
http://www.diabetes.ca

Centers for Disease Control and Prevention, Diabetes Home Page
http://www.cdc.gov/nccdphp

Children with Diabetes
http://www.castleweb.com
Diabetes Care Profile Newsletters
http://www.comed.com.80/novo/profile

Diabetes Interview Newsletter
listserv@netcom.com

The Diabetes Knowledgebase
http://www.biostat.wisc.edu/diaknow/index.htm

Diabetes Mall
http://www.diabetesnet.com

Diabetic Forum
listserv@lehigh.edu

DiNet
http://www.diabetesnet.com/index.html

Food and Drug Administration
http://www.fda.gov

Food and Nutrition Information Center
http://www.nalusda.gov/fnic

International Research Project on Diabetes
listserv@kamikaze.com

Joslin Diabetes Center
http://www.joslin.harvard.edu

Lehigh Diabetic Archives
http://lehigh.edu/lists/diabetic/

Medical Matrix Guide to Internet Resources
http://www.slackinc.com/matrix

Minimed Technologies (manufacturer of insulin pumps)
http://www.minimed.com/.

National Institute of Diabetes and Digestive and Kidney Diseases (NIDDK)
http://www.niddk.nih.gov

Bibliography

Alterman, S. 1996. *How to Control Diabetes: A Complete Guide and Meal Planner to Live a Longer, Healthier, and Happier Life.* Hollywood, Fla.: Lifetime Books.

American Diabetes Association. 1996. *American Diabetes Association Complete Guide to Diabetes.* Alexandria, Va.: American Diabetes Association.

Beaser, R. 1994. *Outsmarting Diabetes: A Dynamic Approach for Reducing the Effects of Insulin-Dependent Diabetes.* Boston: Joslin Diabetes Center.

Beaser, R., and J. V. C. Hill. 1995. *The Joslin Guide to Diabetes: A Program for Managing Your Treatment.* New York: Simon and Schuster.

Biermann, J., and B. Toohey. 1992. *The Diabetic's Total Health Book.* New York: Putnam Publishing Group.

Brody, J. 1985. *Jane Brody's Good Food Cookbook.* New York: W.W. Norton and Co.

Culverwell, M. 1995. "Putting Diabetes on the Map." *JDF International Countdown.* Winter, 28–37.

Dawson, L. 1994. "Diabetes on a Shoestring Budget." *Diabetes Forecast,* November, 29–33.

Dawson, L. 1996. "Progress on the Patch." *Diabetes Forecast,* January, 46(4), 63.

Diabetes Forecast. 1994. "Genetics of Diabetes." *Diabetes Forecast,* July, 58–60.

Diabetes Forecast. 1995. Reader survey. *Diabetes Forecast.* 48/9: 33–37.

Diabetes Interview. 1995. "Company Has $27 Million and a Dream: Less Invasive Testing." *Diabetes Interview,* September, 11.

Diabetes Interview. 1995. "Eye on the Future: Watch Development Progressing Smoothly." *Diabetes Interview,* November, 40.

Dinsmoor, R. S. 1994. "Alternative Medicine, What Works, What Doesn't, and Why." *Diabetes Self-Management,* November/December, 11(5), 6-12.

Dinsmoor, R. S. 1994. "Is Chromium Just for Bumpers? Mineral Supplement Update." *Diabetes Self-Management,* 11(6), 50–54.

Eisenberg, D. M. 1993. "Unconventional Medicine in the United States." *New England Journal of Medicine,* January, 328/4: 246–252.

Elliott, J. 1990. *If Your Child Has Diabetes: An Answer Book for Parents.* New York: Putnam Publishing Group.

Franz, M. 1987. *Exchanges for All Occasions: Meeting the Challenge of Diabetes.* POB 739, Wayzata, MN, 55391: Diabetes Center, Inc.

Gough, D. A., and J. C. Armour. 1995. "Development of the Implantable Glucose Sensor: What Are the Prospects and Why Is It Taking So Long?" *Diabetes,* 44(9), 1005–1009.

Guthrie, D. W., and R. A. Guthrie. *The Diabetes Sourcebook: Today's Methods and Ways to Give Yourself the Best Care.* Los Angeles: RGA Publishing Group.

Jovanovic-Peterson, L., J. Biermann, and B. Toohey. 1996. *The Diabetic Woman.* New York: Putnam Publishing Group.

Jovanovic-Peterson, L., and C. M. Peterson. 1995. *A Touch of Diabetes.* POB 59032, Minneapolis, Minn., 55459: Chronimed Publishing.

Kolata, G. 1998. "U.S. Approves Sale of Impotence Pill; Huge Market Seen." *The New York Times.* March 28, A1.

Lacy, P. E. 1995. "Treating Diabetes with Transplanted Cells." *Scientific American,* July, 50–58.

Lodewick, P. A. 1996. *The Diabetic Man: A Guide to Health and Success.* Los Angeles: Lowell House.

Mirsky, S., and J. R. Heilman. 1981. *Diabetes: Controlling It the Easy Way.* New York: Random House.

Monk, A. 1996. *Managing Type II Diabetes: Your Invitation to a Healthier Lifestyle.* Minneapolis, Minn.: IDC Publishing.

NIDDK. 1996. "NIH Tests Insulin Capsule to Prevent Type I Diabetes." U.S. Department of Health and Human Services, Public Health Service, National Institutes of Health. September 10.

Peragallo-Dittko, V. 1995. "Blood Glucose Meters: A Status Report." *Diabetes Self-Management,* September/October, 12(5), 43–45.

Quickel, K. E. 1996. "Diabetes in a Managed Care System." *Annals of Internal Medicine,* January, 124:1: 2, 160–163.

Ratner, R. E. 1992. "Working Around Employment Discrimination." *Diabetes Self-Management,* January/February, 33–34.

Saudek, C. D. 1993. "Future Developments in Insulin Delivery Systems." *Diabetes Care,* 16(Supplement 3), 122–132.

Starr, B. 1995. "The State of Health Care in America." *Business and Health Magazine,* 13 (Supplement C), 56–60.

Tamborlane, W. V., et al. 1994. "Implications of the DCCT Results in Treating Children and Adolescents with Diabetes." *Clinical Diabetes,* September/October, 12:5, 115.

Tonnessen, D. 1996. *Fifty Essential Things to Do When the Doctor Says It's Diabetes.* New York: Penguin.

University of Miami Diabetes Research Institute. 1996. "University of Miami Diabetes Research Institute Launches Critical Trial, Medical Milestone Achieved." *Miami Medical News,* March 13.

Whitaker, J. M. 1987. *Reversing Diabetes.* New York: Warner Books.

Index

A

B

F

G